GAPS GUIDE:

SIMPLE STEPS TO HEAL BOWELS, BODY, AND BRAIN

2ND EDITION

Author Info & Contact:

Baden D. Lashkov

www.gapsguide.com

Cover design:

Jennifer Poohachoff

Cover image:

Photo by Allan Jenkins

Observer Magazine Organic Allotment

www.guardian.co.uk/lifeandstyle/allotment

Project Management: Skylark Disraeli

Editors: Kristine Thornley, Skylark Disraeli

Proofreaders: Skylark Disraeli, Christine Dudgeon

Indexer: Christine Dudgeon

Layout: Kristine Thornley

TABLE OF CONTENTS

PREFACE

Recently, I was lobbying to a committee for new options for marginalized people. Specifically, I was pitching that the group focus its efforts on increasing marginalized people's access to housing and disability benefits cheques, so that they could rest deeply, and feed themselves food that was healthy for their bodies, rather than the donuts and coffee commonly served at shelters. When I explained that these were the social supports that had helped me, one member looked at me and said, "But, you're different. You're smart, clear, and articulate. That wouldn't work for them."

"No, I'm not different," I replied. "That's my point. If you had seen me years ago, you would have seen one more of 'them.' The only difference is that I've had several years of safe, quiet housing and real food. Give any person on the street the same things, and in a few years you'll see another happy, articulate person in our circle."

This book includes my experience of recovery from "mental" illness. Although every attempt has been made to be as accurate as possible, the account provided is only a general summary. In order to focus on the "how" of recovery, this—and the six other stories of recovery provided within this Guide—are very sparsely told.

INTRODUCTION

Gut and Psychology Syndrome, commonly referred to as "GAPS," is a term used to reflect a state of intestinal bacterial imbalance resulting in any combination of physical, behavioural, emotional, or cognitive symptoms. A program for healing this imbalance proved transformative in the lives of my son and me. Six months after seeing our first results, I started helping other people online—parents doing it for their kids and others doing it for themselves. This publication is the result. The book shares the stories of seven people's recoveries, provides practical steps to the program, incorporates answers to frequently asked questions, and directs you to further resources.

This Guide is intended as a companion to the book *Gut and Psychology Syndrome: Natural Treatments for Dyspraxia, Autism, A.D.D., Dyslexia, A.D.H.D., Depression, and Schizophrenia* by Dr. Natasha Campbell-McBride. This Guide is not a condensation of Dr. Campbell-McBride's book. Rather, it is a complementary work, providing tips for the practical application of the program from a lay person.

Dr. Campbell-McBride read the first edition of *GAPS Guide* before its release and praised it enthusiastically, noting it would be a great help to people accessing it. I was unable to reach Dr. Campbell-McBride to request a pre-read of this edition, so this edition of *GAPS Guide* has not been read in advance by her. As with the first edition, this Guide includes tips, ideas, and perspectives not presented by Dr. Campbell-McBride. Thus, just as with the first edition, not all of this Guide's content is official GAPS information. Again, the content of this Guide has been developed by a lay person as a result of direct, personal experience and four years of dialogue with countless people doing the program. For Dr. Campbell-McBride's direct perspective, always refer to her work or consult directly with Dr. Campbell-McBride.

I strongly recommend that you also read Dr. Campbell-McBride's book and, at least monthly, Dr. Campbell-McBride's regularly updated FAQ document, as presented in a searchable PDF at www.gapsdiet.com/FAQs.html. I also recommend that you join at least one of the free, online GAPS support groups and/or the peer phone support list (offered through the GAPShelp e-mail list). The e-mail support lists often provide quick answers to specific questions not covered here, as well as infuse your changing lifestyle with wonderful support from real people who are on this journey with you. Similarly, the phone support is an invaluable tool for folks who need to hear a reassuring, live voice. These and additional supports, including four lists of health care practitioners familiar with GAPS, are referenced throughout this Guide. All supports mentioned in this paragraph are linked to from the *Support for You* page at GAPSguide.com.

The GAPS program is reported to have resolved symptoms of a number of conditions, including Crohn's disease, colitis, diverticulitis, celiac disease, cystic fibrosis, diarrhea, depression, obsessive compulsive disorder, schizophrenia, attention deficit (with or without hyperactivity) disorder, anxiety, rheumatoid arthritis, autism spectrum disorder, night wakings, eczema, non-anaphylactic allergies, asthma, behavioural problems, learning disabilities, gas, bloating, psoriasis, constipation, feeding difficulties (including "picky eating"), colic, reflux, vomiting, heartburn, dyspraxia, urinary and fecal incontinence, malnutrition, stomach pains, stool abnormalities, autoimmune disorders, and more. Really, GAPS is intended to heal one thing—an imbalance of gut flora—which merely manifests as any or all of the above. For an ever-expanding list of symptoms reported to have been alleviated or resolved through GAPS, please see the *Conditions Addressed* page at GAPSguide.com.

Changes to one's diet, exercise routine, medication or any other factor that influences one's health should be conducted under the direct supervision of a qualified health practitioner. (I am not a health practitioner, so I am not able to provide advice. My presentation is limited to considerations gleaned from personal experience and from experiences reported by others.)

Using this Guide

By the time people are desperate enough to consider changing their eating habits, they are usually already coping with intense symptoms in themselves and/or in their children. They may also have been sleep-deprived for some time. Plus, previous attempts to remedy the issues may have all but swallowed their wallets. For all of these reasons, people coming to the GAPS program tend to be overwhelmed and stressed to the hilt.

This Guide aims to make GAPS as simple as possible. As such, the steps are broken down into three phases:

1. Preparing for GAPS;
2. Doing Intro; and
3. Progressing further.

Before starting any aspect of the program, please read this Guide in its entirety. Details about any given aspect of the program are presented throughout. To be successful on the program with the minimum of frustration, it will be important to have read this entire book through at least once before beginning. Jumping in before reading all of the material presented in this Guide may make your journey more difficult and stressful than necessary.

Also, I suggest keeping a binder of loose-leaf paper by your side while reading the Guide. Jot down any notes—with their associated page numbers for later reference—specific to your circumstances or medical condition. This will help you formulate your personalized program.

Upon reading the entire Guide, please consider starting your journey at the beginning of the *Months 1–3: Preparing for Full GAPS/Intro* section. Some people consider skipping the preparation and/or Intro steps. Their reasons vary: they are coming to GAPS from an already excellent diet, such as one presented by The Weston A. Price Foundation® (WAPF) or the paleolithic/caveman diet communities; they have been ingesting large amounts of probiotic foods for several years; they believe Intro is not important; or they believe Intro will be too hard. Having listened fully to these and many other explanations about why some choose to switch directly and immediately from their current diet to GAPS, or to skip Intro, I continue to strongly recommend a slower, gentler approach, as well as the inclusion of Intro. This noted, the steps you choose are, of course, ultimately up to you.

The approach presented in this Guide is the "safe mode." In other words, what I set forth here assumes you are vulnerable to some of the most common issues. If you have information about yourself that leads you to believe you can or should skip a step or disregard a tip without problems resulting, please feel free to do so.

Again, whether applying the tips presented in this Guide or doing variations, your journey is ideally supported by a health care practitioner, preferably one familiar with GAPS.

The sections *Months 1–3: Preparing for Full GAPS/Intro* and *Months 4–6: GAPS Intro Progression* are each preceded by a suggested timeline (i.e., Months 1–3 and Months 4–6). These are simply to emphasize how much time one might do well to take in reaching and completing each phase. Again, the time you actually spend in each phase will be determined by your personal circumstances and choices.

Finally, within this Guide, I refer regularly to two online resources. Rather than present these two website addresses at every instance, I list them here for you:

1. GAPSguide.com: This Guide's companion website presents recipes, tips, lists of practitioners familiar with GAPS, and so on. All of these are linked

to from the website's *Support for You* page found at http://gapsguide.com/about/support/.

2. The Frequently Asked Questions (FAQ) document compiled by Dr. Campbell-McBride. This resource is regularly updated and provides details not covered in Dr. Campbell-McBride's book, *Gut and Psychology Syndrome*, plus answers to questions submitted to her, program modifications for specific medical conditions, new additions to the list of recommended foods, and so on. Updated as often as once a month, this important document is presented as a searchable PDF at www.gapsdiet.com/FAQs.html. I strongly recommend that you read the entire paper through once, preferably immediately upon finishing your first read of *GAPS Guide*, and then read the subsequent updates (as presented at the top of the document) as they are added every month or so.

Our Stories

I was an intensely shy child—really, a walking anxiety attack. It showed in my fingernails, bitten to the quick from a young age, a habit that would defy all remedies. Stomach aches were almost constant. From the age of four, I felt chokingly bewildered as to where and how I fit in (for years I wondered if I were an alien!). My vague but deep fear resulted in my being late for school so many times that, when I was finally on time, my second grade teacher had the entire class stand up and applaud!

Earaches and ear infections were common for me. My feet hurt constantly. I ground my teeth to the point that my jaw ached terribly. I was chronically overstimulated, overwhelmed, and depressed. The first suicidal thoughts I clearly recall occurred at nine years of age; they persisted into adulthood.

As a teenager, my periods brought unbearable back pain—I fantasized about climbing into my family's deep freezer to relieve it. I developed cystic acne across my face, neck, shoulders, and back. My hair was dulling; some turned grey. Always a picky eater, my habits worsened as I grew. By age 14, I had sworn off meat, and my "meals" were made up of white pasta, canned tomato sauce, cheese, some fruit, and copious chocolate bars. My system couldn't take much more abuse and a trauma at summer camp triggered persistent self-harm: to experience even transient relief from overwhelming psychological pain, I began cutting myself and bashing my head on sinks and walls. My high school's environment, including bullying to the degree of threats on my life, finally tipped the scales—under stress, I would hallucinate or pass out.

In grade 12, I made the decision to save my own life. I dropped out of school, took an apartment, and opened a second-hand shop. This new lifestyle suited me well. Although still struggling with anxiety and depression, and generally unable to manage the functions involved in cooking and driving, I coasted along relatively well for some time. At age 19, I moved to another city and started caring for seniors. Again, these changes proved very healthy and I functioned somewhat well for several years. At 22, however, I was working split shifts in home support and residential care, volunteering 25 hours per week, and eating very poorly. I couldn't fathom why after eating an entire pot of pasta, I would still feel ravenous. During this period I lost my sight several times for up to a minute each time. My energy was supported by an instant chocolate-coffee drink and the cookies my clients and employers fed me.

Eventually I crashed. I suffered a complete physical and mental breakdown. My heart raced. I was exhausted but I couldn't sleep. My hands trembled almost constantly, and from one moment to the next I transitioned involuntarily from over-the-top laughter to deep sadness and weeping. I developed severe, bleeding eczema. Much of the time, my physical senses were heightened to a painful degree. At times, a strong stutter overtook my speech. I also experienced "verbal dyslexia." For example, regardless of how hard I focused, when I tried to say "mac," it would come out as "cam." I struggled to cover these bizarre episodes, but some proved bigger challenges to hide. For example, mere blocks from my home, panic would build in my heart as I would suddenly not remember where I lived or how to get there.

I had always been a compassionate person, but now I felt waves of rage. My body was screaming at me as it shut down, but I could not comprehend what was happening or why. Finally unable to work, I returned to my hometown, where I lived off of my savings until those were exhausted and I was left with little choice but to apply for welfare. At one point I was so sick I couldn't stand long enough to shower, nor lift my hands above my head long enough to wash my hair. After sitting in a bath, I would climb out, panting, then lie on the mat and sleep until I could muster up enough energy to move out of the bathroom. My family brought me my grocery orders: white pasta, lentils, and kegs of apple juice. One day, I was not able to press the tab on the juice keg hard enough to release any of its contents. Still unaware of the depth of my debilitation, I assumed the keg was broken and asked my dad to return it to the store. The moment he tested it—with success—was a defining one for me: I was weaker than a toddler.

Depression took a firmer grip. I would channel all my energy into an hour or two out with friends, then come home to complete collapse and despair. Eventually, with no intervention other than rest, my body did rebuild some strength. My confidence shattered, I entered a work training program. Determined to find my way back to a "normal" life, I rode my bicycle uphill six kilometres, worked in construction and landscaping for eight hours, coasted home, carried my bike up three flights of stairs, then crashed in my hallway, sleeping there with my boots on. My progress during the program gave me hope, but once independent of its supportive environment, my success didn't last long.

I continued to experience extreme sensitivity to ambient heat and cold. In our summer's scorching temperatures, my nose would suddenly start bleeding. In the winter, even indoors I would layer on long johns, one or more sweaters, a winter coat, and a wool hat, and then set myself in a small room with a heater on full blast—and still shiver. Out in a park, I could not relax and enjoy an expanse of lush green field because I was acutely aware of every individual blade of grass, and I felt overwhelmed and panicky by this. My sense of time was skewed: often I would believe several days had passed when only a handful of hours had. Intense fear and a general sense of shame prevented me from completing simple tasks, such as making a purchase, in front of others. Poor auditory processing meant that using a phone was stressful and futile, at best. I often could not manage the executive functions involved in driving; at the same time, I could not cope with going more than one direction from home in a given day, so I had to schedule my activities to head only east (then home) one day, and west (then home) the next. Often my brain would simply "shut down," at which times I could not think, respond, speak, or act. What I could do in those moments was recognize that I wasn't functioning, thus feel terrified. Sleep was sporadic. Although desperate for rest, I would often be awake for up to 36 hours, finally fall asleep for two or three hours, then wake again.

The next several years brought countless hospitalizations and psychiatric out-patient programs. I would eventually have a range of diagnoses—one for every doctor I had seen. Doctors prescribed major tranquilizers, minor tranquilizers, lithium, and antidepressants. For the most part, I declined them. I wanted to maintain the tiny bit of control I had left and, ironically for a suicidal person, I didn't want to "give up." I viewed the taking of drugs as doing exactly that, as conceding defeat to symptoms while also resigning myself to a lifetime of them.

Further, I could not stand the thought of adding permanent tardive dyskinesia,[1] for example, to my list of issues. Utterly unable to cope with roommates or family, I ate in soup kitchens and slept in shelters, on the streets, or in low-cost rooms while perpetually trying to return to work.

A normal life, however, seemed further and further from ever being possible. I wasn't getting better, and now I was sharing accommodations with up to two hundred men, showering semi-publicly, and eating mush shoulder-to-shoulder with people horking, hacking, and threatening. I couldn't stand it any longer. I worked up the courage to ask my family to support my suicide. Instead, my mum prayed. Shortly after, a friend asked me to do one more thing before making the ultimate decision: see Dr. Abram Hoffer. I was certain the last thing I needed was another psychiatrist. (The most recent in a long line, an "expert" who had been flown in to review my case, had spoken with me for just ten minutes before determining me "fine." Despite my severe symptoms, he ordered that my lithium be abruptly stopped and my hospitalization ended.) But, what did I have to lose? Suicide at 3:00 instead of at 1:00? I could do that.

Dr. Hoffer was a mild, gentle character. Some of his first words to me were: "You're not crazy. You have a biochemical disorder." His words were like spring rain. In a sense, I had already known I wasn't "crazy," because by this point I was aware that no one was. I had experienced what I had, and I had witnessed similar challenges in countless street friends. I knew these people, and I was keenly aware that they were, for the most part, sound, intelligent, sensible people for whom medical issues had cost them their jobs, then their homes, and then their welfare cheques. But what on earth did he mean by "biochemical disorder?"

Dr. Hoffer taught me the most basic and important of concepts: the brain is an organ. (Sounds obvious, doesn't it? Indeed. So why do so many still view the brain as something we can control with "good intention and strong will" any more than we can the pancreas or the heart?) Initially a chemist, Dr. Hoffer's work led him to psychiatry where he applied the principles of chemistry to human health. Using diet and vitamins, as well as medications as needed in the interim, he successfully treated countless people for a constellation of symptoms now often diagnosed as high-functioning autism, social learning disabilities, personality disorders, schizophrenia (not to be confused with dissociative disorder or "split personality"), bipolar disorder, and generalized anxiety disorder—in other words, any complex health picture involving symptoms such as depression, fear,

---

[1] Involuntary movements sometimes triggered by some psychiatric medications.

heightened senses, confusion, difficulty in understanding or expressing, hallucinations, and so on.

The causes of these symptoms continue to be hotly debated, but Dr. Hoffer's perspective was that these issues derive from deficiencies in key vitamins and minerals, and are often exacerbated by stress. As Dr. Hoffer explained, behaviour that responds to stimuli is not "crazy" at all; rather, it is deeply sane. In other words, if you saw a five-tonne elephant charging at you, you'd run, too! A body out of whack may tell the eyes that a five-tonne elephant is charging, or tell the ears that one's name is being said on the news. The "sane" response to the charging elephant is to run. The "sane" response to your name being said on the news is to shush everyone around you, listen closely, and become downright indignant at the misrepresentation! Likewise, when you look up from this book and see the wall across from you, you assume the wall is really there. Because you can see it, it is rational to believe the wall is indeed there and to respond accordingly (i.e., not walk into it). Accordingly, behaviour one might view as "crazy" is not—it is a natural and appropriate response to the input one's body is feeding his brain.

Immediately following my first appointment with Dr. Hoffer, a new friend who had previously "gone the journey" from debilitating depression to outstanding health took me into his home for a week and guided me through a basic allergen-elimination diet, as recommended by Dr. Hoffer. Between the medication, vitamins, and diet prescribed by Dr. Hoffer, I was happy and working again within a week. Through methodical testing (reintroducing foods one at a time), I discovered that if I ate lentils, I became so weak that I could neither stand nor lift my arms, and that if I ate chocolate, I became overwhelmed with anger and violent energy. With a sound diet in place, I was quickly able to eliminate the medication. As long as I stuck with the diet, my health was good. Indeed, I was one of the many people for whom Dr. Hoffer's program was incredibly successful.

Around that time, a social worker noted to me that, in her experience, those following Dr. Hoffer's diet and vitamin recommendations did indeed see success. She stated sadly that many patients chose to do the vitamins alone, ignoring the dietary aspect, and consequently saw limited results. Unfortunately, this is common in our culture. Most of us want 20 years of toxicity reversed with a pill while vehemently rejecting the notion that other items we put into our mouths could be an issue!

Alas, I was only one step ahead of that mindset. My experience with Dr. Hoffer's protocol made it clear to me that I needed to maintain a strict diet. That didn't mean I did it, though. Despite my results, I eventually returned to junk food and my other intolerances. My desperate hospitalizations resumed.

I relocated yet again. My newest doctor, Dr. Jim Howie, proved utterly supportive through all my subsequent efforts toward healing, including my attempts to return to nutrition. (I will never forget "meeting" him. In a bout of severe dysphoria, I was sobbing so hard I was, despite my best intentions and effort, completely unable to look up. For the duration of our first interaction, I saw only his shoes!) Eventually, I committed to a one-year course of the antidepressant, Paxil®. All things considered, this was a good move. Although my level of sensitivity allowed me to take only one-quarter of what was considered a "minimum dose," the drug worked wonders. My brain was finally quiet. On the medication, my obsessive compulsive disorder (OCD) and anxiety largely resolved, thus depression and hallucinations were pre-empted. My body also began responding normally to heat and cold. Most importantly, I was able to do practical things like shop for food, as well as attend therapy and apply what I was learning. After a year, I was able to gently wean off Paxil®. With the continued support of therapy, I established a low-key lifestyle in which self-care and healing were prioritized. I still struggled with a variety of issues, but the extremes which had been driving me to consider suicide were, thankfully, over. Around this time, I started volunteering in a field that was well-served by my life experience. For the four years that our work was funded, I gained confidence and skills in a flexible, supportive environment. My detail-oriented, endlessly active mind finally had a positive outlet! Because the work was largely solitary and electronic, my disability did not severely interfere. As a result, although still dealing with some degree of illness, I felt greatly fulfilled and blessed.

When the contract ended, I felt a deep sense of loss, but I soon received the happy news that I was pregnant. My history had demonstrated clearly to me the impact of nutrition, so from the day of conception, I began taking a quality prenatal vitamin and eating an all-organic diet rich in vegetables and other whole foods. And then I threw them all up—every day, all day, for several weeks. As it turned out, my best efforts were working against me: the iron in the prenatal pill was ultimately determined to be the trigger for my profuse vomiting. Even after that discovery, it wasn't smooth sailing. I bled regularly. I had miscarried in the past, so I was deeply concerned. This combined with other stresses ultimately overwhelmed me, and to my primarily ovo-lacto vegetarian diet I added daily helpings of Twinkies, chips, pop, and candy. Those were about the extent of my toxins. I steered clear of cigarette smoke, did not drink coffee, and did not use drugs (prescription or otherwise). I even wore a mask while gardening to ensure no possible transmission of toxoplasmosis! I made every effort to keep the pregnancy as low-stress and viable as possible. Despite all my precautions, my son was born six weeks prematurely.

From birth, my son had many challenges: he struggled both to breathe and to coordinate the reflexes involved in eating. At some points, if he were not held every moment of the day and night he would scream. For his first two years, he was unable to eat anything except breast milk. In all but a few instances, if other food even touched his lips, he would vomit. He was severely iron deficient. Throughout each night, he woke at least every two to four hours. He ground his teeth so hard that people across the room would ask what the bizarre noise was. His brand new teeth rapidly disintegrated, but his severe oral aversion prevented our regular dentist from providing treatment. (Luckily, one of our support workers referred us to a dentist specializing in treatment for people with issues like my son had. Between the competent and professional actions of this dentist and the dental surgeon she quickly referred us to, his teeth were saved just before surgical extraction would otherwise have occurred.) His language was severely delayed: he had no words at all for his first two years. As a result of this and his lack of consistent response to people speaking to him, support workers urged me to have his hearing tested. I was confident it was fine—I knew his hearing to be quite sensitive and he had never had so much as an ear infection. Hearing impairment was indeed ruled out. These challenges had a different, but as yet unknown, cause.

In seemingly random moments, my son would suddenly begin snaking backwards across the floor on his belly, screaming, finally pressing his forehead against a wall (usually in a closet) or hiding under blankets, terror in his eyes. At these times, it seemed he did not recognize me, and he found no comfort in my efforts to soothe him. Other times, such as when more than one person was singing, he would suddenly begin bashing his head on the floor. He could not tolerate baths, haircuts, or toothbrushing. He ran vigorously toward traffic. Much of the time, his belly was distended. Incontinent, he was unable to potty train. He stopped growing: Over the course of one year, his height dropped from the fiftieth percentile to the second.

Speech and occupational therapists came regularly to assess him, teach him new skills, attempt to get him more comfortable with eating, and train his caregivers in interventions. We made little gain. When parents of children the same age or older would exclaim, "Isn't it amazing how they change in their second year? They become completely different people! One day they have no language, and the next they're babbling non-stop and you're having conversations!" I would smile and nod, but feel a tight knot of fear in my belly: *Why wasn't my son doing any of that?*

Our pediatrician conducted multiple tests to determine what might be interfering with my son's development. Besides his low iron, everything appeared to be fine internally. He was well-supported by my breast milk (my own body, on the other hand, was struggling under the impact of being the sole source of food for a very heavy and active toddler). Ultimately, our pediatrician was at a loss to explain or remedy the issues, but she continued to be a valued support and kept us bolstered.

Happily, one random day after his second birthday, my son ate. From that point, he quickly progressed through the stages of mushy, chunky, and solids. He also started to speak one and two words at a time. We were elated! Although the challenging behaviours continued, we focused on enjoying the gains he was making. Shortly after his third birthday, however, he developed chronic diarrhea. On the basis of the newest symptom, our general physician suggested my son might have celiac disease, and advised that I try dietary interventions. When I researched celiac disease, I learned that most of my son's symptoms—missing tooth enamel, iron deficiency, behavioural issues, developmental delays, halted growth, and diarrhea—were addressed by that single diagnosis. Online, I located two dietary options proposed for celiac disease. One, a gluten-free diet, would be relatively easy to achieve but would require lifelong adherence to maintain even its limited results. The other, the Specific Carbohydrate Diet (SCD), was a diet temporarily more restricted, thus more challenging to implement, but reportedly it could actually heal the gut, ultimately allowing for a wide range of healthy foods to be eaten. One website claimed that both celiac disease and autistic symptoms could be relieved by the latter—the promise of addressing the full range of my son's issues was the clincher.

We didn't implement the SCD right away; the first step in our dietary transition involved simply pulling out many common allergens. On Day 1 of our initial attempt at an elimination diet, my son slept through the night for the first time in his life! The next day, he had a normal stool for the first time in six weeks. Food was clearly an issue. Over the subsequent weeks, I experimented, observed, studied, and experimented again. We saw that his symptoms worsened with many foods and improved with others. As I continued to transition him to the SCD, he initially protested with tantrums and tears over the withdrawal of cow's milk and the processed cookies he was used to having every afternoon, but he also welcomed all the new foods (including copious SCD desserts) that we put in front of him. Much to my amazement, he soon spoke his first sentence, and from that point on he spoke freely (albeit often haltingly). That same week, he also potty trained himself. His fear of bathing also disappeared—he requested a bath, got in happily, and played in it gleefully for hours. His oral aversion resolved completely—from his very next dental appointment he enjoyed even his dental cleanings! His language, cognition, and physical development continued to show great gains. My son became, for the most part, relaxed, calm, easygoing, tremendously happy, and highly sociable. However, even when we were doing things "perfectly," we did experience ups and downs, with some of the initial symptoms recurring (especially sleep disturbances and loose stools). That is, although the consistency and colour of his stools remained markedly improved, they also continued to be "all over the map" for the first several months of healing. Mostly the major stool issues—as well as the most concerning of his earlier behaviours—returned only when he had a virus, tried a food that proved too advanced for his system to handle, or consumed too much fruit in a day.

After supporting my son with the SCD for four months, we made a trip to see an established naturopath, in hopes he would tell us that other foods could be included earlier than the SCD protocol proposed. I had brought enough SCD food to last the four days we would be away from home. However, I was unaware that the almond bread needed to be refrigerated, so it rapidly turned mouldy. This meant we went through our homemade yogurt much more quickly than planned. Far from home and at a complete loss, I fed my son things I hoped were "close enough"—specifically, whole nuts, commercial yogurt, and bread made with sprouted grains—and hoped for the best. He regressed horribly. No longer used to his old symptoms, I broke too.

As it happens, I was reading the book *Gut and Psychology Syndrome*, by Dr. Natasha Campbell-McBride. In her book, Dr. Campbell-McBride presented a syndrome and a healing program both commonly referred to as "GAPS." Its diet was largely based on the SCD. It was obvious to me that I needed to get my son back onto the diet that had resolved so many of his symptoms, but this book made it clear that I should be on it, too. Although most of my issues were now "mild" in comparison to what I had been through earlier in life, parenting (especially considering the circumstances) was challenging all the gains I had made. Further, the foot pain I had always experienced had recently intensified, leaving me at one point unable to walk for three days. Also, some time after my son's birth, my periods—which previously had involved "merely" severe back pain—had become very intense and frightening. A day or so before each one, I would be overcome with weakness, my legs would give out, my skin would become very pale, and my lips would take on a distinctly blue tinge. Because this issue had quickly resolved on the "mostly SCD" I had been doing in tandem with my son's diet, and because of the results I had experienced years earlier on Dr. Hoffer's very similar program, I knew my body responded well to this approach. I had been focused entirely on my son, but clearly my own health demanded intervention, too.

In a major regression, the SCD protocol is to return briefly to its introductory phase. Since I had regularly been eating non-SCD when outside of the house, I would need to start there too. I started us both over, but this time with the GAPS introductory protocol. On this and the complete GAPS program, we saw improvements even beyond those achieved on the SCD alone. Temporary setbacks and our inherent genetic disabilities notwithstanding, my son and I have become very well.

It boggles my mind every single day that something so simple (so to speak) could bring about such tremendous changes. We aren't perfect, of course, nor are we superhuman, but my son and I are healthy and happy to a degree I once would not have even felt able to hope for.

For me, the combination of GAPS' food, ferments, baths, and rest virtually eliminated my anxiety, free-floating fears, and depression. Six weeks into the program, I realized that a severe obsessive–compulsive pattern had disappeared. (As with my son, a virus or a period of intense healing can trigger some degree of these, but only fleetingly.) I found myself speaking more honestly and freely than ever before. My self-esteem blossomed. My thinking was vastly clearer, and my planning more calm and logical. My emotional capacities and tolerances increased. Several intense, lifelong food phobias resolved. I no longer experienced heartburn after eating raw garlic or raw onions. A patch of severe eczema, which had developed then disappeared long before GAPS, resurfaced during healing then resolved completely. I started sleeping through most nights. The menstrual issues and foot pain were also eliminated.

Likewise, the vast majority of my son's original issues remain resolved. He talks, dresses himself, bathes, eats well, plays, and socializes. From a medical point of view, concerns about my son have been drastically downgraded. Although most issues resolved, some aspects have persisted (e.g., fatigue with writing and some difficulty reading social cues), but his cheerfulness, kindness, groundedness, and general enthusiasm for life are profound and obvious. Bedwetting and sleep disturbances ebb and flow in direct relation to a number of factors. Eliminating oxalates from his GAPS diet showed promising results in these areas, but at the time of this writing, we are choosing to test the effects of other approaches for these issues.

Of note is that our outstanding results were achieved even upon implementing less than 100% of the program! That is, over the course of 2½ years we ate only GAPS foods, completed the full Intro progression several times, committed ourselves more and more deeply to an eco-friendlier, lower-stress lifestyle, and took regular detox baths. However, over the same period we rarely remembered the bottled oils; we juiced for only about one week before I let go of the juicing cost, process, and mess; we did not manage to incorporate organ foods (but we have since begun to do so randomly); and outside of each round of Intro, we had broth one to three times per week at most. And our results were excellent. Of course, I have to wonder what our results would have been had we followed the program 100%. We didn't because the amount we did was as much as I could manage as a sole, working parent with her own disabilities. But I'm not merely satisfied with our results—I'm overjoyed! By doing even most of the program, our lives were changed dramatically for the good.

With our bodies no longer consumed with the task of mere survival, and with good health in place, we have been able to begin moving on to secondary therapies, learning that which we never had a chance to before. For me, this involves learning new relaxation and relational approaches, among other things. For my son, it means learning to read social cues more effectively, improving his muscle tone, and facilitating deeper self-regulation.

I firmly believe that even after healing, a nutrient-dense diet free of processed food and limited in starches is ideal. This noted, 2½ years after we began our SCD/GAPS journey, I started introducing non-GAPS items into our lives. Since then, my son and I have moved in and out of Full GAPS as our health or other circumstances dictate. For example, when two more children—little ones totally unused to and fearful of dense nutrition—came into our lives, I opted to adjust the diet of my son and I to one equivalent to that presented under this Guide's section *Months 1–3: Preparing for Full GAPS/Intro.* That is, I adjusted our diet to one incorporating as much GAPS food as I felt was necessary in the new circumstance, while allowing other ones to serve as transitional foods.

My son, now eight years old, gets a kick out of being allowed to sometimes eat anything from starches to non-foods. (I do, too, but personally I find it much easier and more beneficial to live within the clear parameters of Full GAPS, rather than re-trigger—then attempt to manage—the cravings that come with ingestion of starches.) Unlike at the beginning of our journey, when even a teaspoon of fruit would trigger screaming and flailing in my son, neither of us shows immediate negative consequences to any non-GAPS food. We both, though, experience a very obvious resurfacing of symptoms if we eat too many of these too often. I find it takes only a few days of excess conventional food for me to feel unwell. Happily, I also find it only takes three to seven days on GAPS to re-establish feelings of well-being. I regularly reset our bodies by doing Stage 1 for a few days, doing the complete Intro progression again, or even by just returning to Full GAPS for a stretch of time.

I estimate that over the course of most weeks, approximately 95% of our diet is GAPS, while the other 5% involves other foods, including the most processed of options. (A major boon for us has been the option to include commercial—albeit grass-fed and organic—whey powder. This blended with canned coconut milk, coconut oil, frozen banana chunks, salt, and vanilla or raw cocoa results in a portable power shake that has done my son a world of good in terms of energy, calm, and satiation.) We eat and drink fermented foods regularly, and also take commercial probiotic capsules randomly. We do courses of *Saccharomyces boulardii*, and experiment with additional approaches such as commercial cleanses for parasites or the liver. I continue to hope that at some point I'll muster the organizational "oomph" to include a daily dose of each of the three GAPS-recommended oils.

Some weeks we make more exceptions and some weeks we make fewer. Every experiment gives us additional information about what our bodies can and cannot tolerate, and about how lackadaisical we can and cannot be. (I regularly share the results and new awareness in my blog posts on the GAPSguide.com website.) But even if I were to snarf down several Twinkies every day from this point forward—thus making myself chronically ill again—and offer my son a similar option, it wouldn't change the fact that returning to my ancestors' traditions has already proven itself capable of bringing both my son and me freedom from symptoms, plus health and happiness. This knowledge gives me much relief, as well as optimism for all others experiencing similarly devastating symptoms.

Two full years after having completed our GAPS program, I note that some things changed for me with GAPS and some did not. I am still essentially an introvert, preferring many hours of quiet and solitude, and I remain constitutionally sensitive, enjoying rest and reading over an athletic lifestyle (although I do enjoy movement). I'm much, much happier. I have more calm and more energy. I'm more focused. I did not become a sourdough-bread-making, garden-growing, radish-pickling Mama like some of the GAPSters I most admire have. I do take much better care of myself, having become aware—through GAPS—of both the positive and negative effects that any given food, belief, relationship, community, or exercise can have on me.

When I go through a phase of eating too little nutrient-dense food, or too much conventional food, I experience mild effects. If I continue further down that path, the effects become moderate, and I happily return to GAPS. Often I judge my post-GAPS lifestyle as being too far removed from the program which changed so much for my son and me, but when I see the pantries of dear friends and neighbours, I realize with a start how even my post-GAPS diet is still actually leagues beyond my pre-GAPS diet and any conventional one! I laugh to realize that my kitchen is still very much a GAPS one.

Every time I have my menstrual period, I feel immensely grateful, remembering where my journey started and what gains I have experienced. The perfectionist in me is keen to maintain a "pure" lifestyle free of any direct toxin, but a strict approach is no longer necessary. I am profoundly glad that I committed to GAPS for 2½ years, and accept that we can now incorporate post-GAPS elements, such as swims in a chlorinated pool during Canada's cold winters, use of a commercial (albeit relatively natural) shampoo when that's more convenient than an egg yolk, or varying amounts of non-GAPS food.

My hope is that in sharing the details of our stories, the recommendations of the GAPS program, and the tips gleaned from personal experience and conversations with countless others live and online, that relief and hope will be yours to experience, too. I'm confident it can be.

I am not a health practitioner. Rather, from our rich range of experience I offer practical ideas about doing GAPS in the situations of: sole parent; low income; blended families with two custodial parents offering vastly different diets; house moves; homeschooling; conventional schooling; full-time work outside of the home; home-based work; person with disabilities; and more. My hope is that by sharing the challenges I have faced and overcome, you will be supported in your path toward increased health for yourself and your loved ones.

CHAPTER 1

THE GAPS PROGRAM

Note: For simplicity's sake, in this book the acronym "GAPS" refers both to the symptoms in need of healing and the healing program itself.

A Brief Overview

GAPS is based on the premise that a healthy balance of gut bacteria serves to protect and, indirectly, nourish the body. When the bacterial field becomes imbalanced, one of our first lines of defence becomes ineffective. Without protection, the gut wall is open to anything that comes along, including fungi, viruses, environmental toxins, and parasites. Also, because food depends on bacteria for its processing, when the balance is off, nutrients cannot be effectively accessed, never mind distributed throughout the body.

This is a very brief explanation of an intricately involved process. For a detailed explanation with helpful illustrations, please see the book *Gut and Psychology Syndrome: Natural Treatments for Dyspraxia, Autism, A.D.D., Dyslexia, A.D.H.D., Depression, and Schizophrenia* by neurologist and nutritionist, Dr. Natasha Campbell-McBride.

Treatment for the syndrome allows the gut lining to heal, restores the correct balance of intestinal bacteria, and relieves the body of an excessive toxic load. These adjustments alleviate symptoms while allowing the digestive system to fully utilize and distribute necessary nutrients so that normal function of all body parts (brain included) can occur.

What causes an imbalance of gut flora? No one thing will do it on its own. Contributing factors include diet, antibiotics, environmental toxins (e.g., lead, mercury, pollution, and chlorine), contraceptive pills, other medications, steroids, and stress. An imbalance in the pregnant mother's gut flora can affect the baby (e.g., when the child comes through the birth canal, his system is filled with an imbalance of flora), and compromised breast milk may offer limited benefits in terms of probiotics. Granted, we live in a world that includes environmental toxins and stress, and antibiotics do have their place. The GAPS program does not propose that you quit work, become a recluse, and live in a yurt (unless you want to!). It's all about your total toxic load. Select your toxins consciously and move them out regularly. For example, is it really necessary to replace your carpets this year? Is pesticide-free food an option for your family? Cleaning with vinegar and baking soda can achieve tremendous results throughout the house without putting your family at risk with harsh cleaning chemicals. Is your illness so severe that it calls for antibiotics, or will rest and ginger tea do the trick?

Regardless of the origin of one's gut imbalance, in the GAPS healing program we aim to address it by (1) sealing the gut wall, (2) rebuilding the body's natural detoxification system so that it can effectively release toxins day after day, and (3) bringing bacteria and yeasts to an optimal balance in the ideal locations for each type. GAPS recognizes that every type of bacteria and yeast has a positive role in its optimal locations and numbers. Every microbe is simply seeking its ideal conditions, as determined by acidity levels, temperature, presence of other bacteria, and so on. Through GAPS, we create in our gut the conditions in which specific bacteria thrive, while the rest stay in their optimal balance in their own ideal locations. One way in which we do this is by taking in only the types of foods even a compromised gut can quickly and thoroughly break down, leaving no remnants to act as food for microbes that would otherwise overwhelm the gut and break down the gut lining. Microbes that do not belong in the gut, or which should not exist in such high proportions there, reduce in number or completely die away from that location. However, they will continue their positive roles in the locations and/or numbers that are correct for them.

This process of balancing microbes and rebuilding the body's natural detoxification system takes time. For most people, a minimum of 18–24 months will be required. The exact timeline will be different for everyone, because it depends on one's age, degree of illness, adherence to the program, number of recommendations incorporated, and the individual body's ability to cope with detoxification. In general, a person should stay on the program for 6–12 months after the last symptom has reared its ugly head (after the initial two years, if any symptoms are persisting, one may at that point consider incorporating additional intensive therapies, such as specific chelation approaches as presented by Dr. Campbell-McBride in her FAQ document).

Many choose to stay on GAPS for many more months or years because they are enjoying it and are continuing to see improvements in their health. Once your gut has healed, chances are very high that you will be able to incorporate other quality foods, such as potatoes or sourdough bread, into your weekly diet. You will also likely be able to get away with eating anything you wish on occasion. Once strengthened, your body will be able to process and eliminate the toxins without noticeable stress. Hopefully, you will not revert back to a conventional diet because that would create toxic overload again.

For most people, once the benefits and deliciousness of GAPS are experienced directly, the duration of the journey becomes a non-issue.

The Program

Often erroneously referred to as "a diet," GAPS is actually a three-part program:

1. Diet,
2. Detoxification, and
3. Supplementation.

Each of these aspects is discussed in detail in the pages that follow.

CHAPTER 2

DIET

The diet part of the GAPS program is essentially the Specific Carbohydrate Diet (SCD). The SCD is a temporary diet of super digestible foods (mostly monosaccharides that do not require complex processes for digestion). It was originally developed by Dr. Sidney V. Haas and Dr. Merrill P. Haas. This father-and-son team developed a protocol, based on several years of successful clinical experience with hundreds of patients, for healing bowel disorders such as celiac disease. Symptoms now categorized under the labels "autism," "pervasive developmental delay," "anxiety," and so on were also found to be addressed.

In 1958, a meeting between Dr. Sidney Haas, Dr. Merrill Haas, and a mother of a very ill child took place. Three years earlier, Elaine Gottschall's daughter, Judy, had been diagnosed with "incurable ulcerative colitis." Several years of mainstream medical treatment had been unsuccessful. Judy's condition had continued to deteriorate and surgery seemed necessary and imminent. However, on the SCD, Judy's symptoms quickly let up. Within two years of implementing the Haas' program, little Judy was symptom-free. Reportedly, she has remained healthy ever since.

The results of this simple approach heavily influenced every subsequent day of Elaine Gottschall's life. Determined to understand more, she completed studies in biochemistry and conducted years of formal research before compiling her book, *Breaking the Vicious Cycle: Intestinal Health Through Diet*. Right up until her death at age 84, Ms. Gottschall continued pursuing answers, while also assisting people from all over the globe to implement the diet.

As a result of Ms. Gottschall's work, several websites, online support groups, and recipe books cropped up, each of which further supported people to implement the lifestyle changes inherent to the SCD. One of the many individuals positively impacted by Ms. Gottschall's work was Dr. Natasha Campbell-McBride. Dr. Campbell-McBride is a neurologist, but when her son developed autism, her extensive medical training was unable to help him. Determined to ease her son's challenges, Dr. Campbell-McBride pursued alternative streams of healing—and found success. Through diet and the ingestion of friendly bacteria, Dr. Campbell-McBride's son became a healthy, fully integrated young man.

In the process of healing her son and patients, Dr. Campbell-McBride developed a three-part program for maximum healing, with an emphasis on behavioural, cognitive, and mood disorders. She tweaked the Specific Carbohydrate Diet for even better results in these areas, established a gentle-yet-effective detoxification protocol, and identified supplements to support both gut and brain function. This became the GAPS healing protocol.

The first priority of GAPS is to clean up and heal the digestive system so that it ceases to be the body's primary source of toxicity, and instead becomes the source of nourishment it is intended to be. The second priority is to remove the toxins that have gathered throughout the body during one's lifetime.

A list of recommended foods is included in this Guide. However, please note that not all GAPS-recommended foods are immediately digestible. For example, as healthy as they are, leafy greens may be very hard on a compromised system. By starting with only the most digestible items, such as well-cooked, non-fibrous vegetables in meat broth, one's gut begins to heal and rebuild, allowing for the reintroduction of raw produce. I recommend that a person move through the steps in the order presented in this Guide: one to three months preparing for GAPS, approximately one month of Full GAPS, then Intro, then at least 18–24 months on Full GAPS before testing additional foods.

What to Eat and When

What Will I Eat?

Pizza, ice cream, stews, pie, brownies, breads, quiche, crackers, puddings, omelettes, curries, risotto, toast, frittata, fruit, baba ghanoush, mashed "potatoes," pancakes and waffles with jam, nuts, "ants on a log," fish, burgers…the list goes on and on!

A GAPS meal can be simple or fancy, raw or cooked, vegan or meaty, light or rich, quick or involved, low-budget or extravagant. Practically any conventional recipe can be transposed into a GAPS one, plus there are several books devoted to SCD or GAPS recipes, and literally hundreds more recipes online. The October 2008 edition of *Canadian Living* magazine claimed that children with celiac disease "can't eat birthday cake, sandwiches, pizza, or hot dog buns." My son's fourth birthday party alone would set this unfortunate rumour to rest!

Breakfast

My son and I eat the same types of things for breakfast as we do for lunch or supper: soup; any style of eggs; stews; casserole; frittata; chicken cold from the fridge; stir-fry; a giant salad with sauerkraut and cubed cheddar mixed in; slices of cheese dipped in guacamole or salsa; salmon patties piled high with fermented vegetables, leafy greens, cucumber slices, salsa, sour cream, and grated cheese; grated cauliflower sautéed in oil and spices; and so on. This morning we reheated and enjoyed leftovers from last night's supper: a multi-meat and veggie stir-fry.

Occasionally, we have pancakes, nuts, fruit, or a smoothie for breakfast, but the vast majority of our breakfasts are eggs, meat, or fish with veggies and a ferment. In the morning, I have more energy for meal preparation—often a casserole is being pulled from the oven well before 10 AM and this becomes our first meal. We both do best starting the day with a warm, grounding, satiating meal.

Lunch

If we will be home for lunch, the information under *Breakfast* applies. If we're going to be away from home during lunch, we fill a pre-conditioned insulated food container with any one of a number of options, including any of the breakfast foods listed above (e.g., eggs, stir-fry, casserole, or soup) or anything leftover from a previous meal. A tuna salad travels well, as does a jar of nut butter with several sticks of celery. Alternatively, we'll carry a can of salmon (with a can opener and spoon), and a whole cucumber, tomato, or bell pepper. We eat these vegetables the same way most people eat apples (i.e., whole and held in the hand). On a hot day, sugars serve rather than deplete us (as they might on a cooler or less active day). On these occasions we might enhance our lunch with whole fruit, or with a homemade fruit smoothie carried in a cold-conditioned insulated food container.

During Intro's earliest stages, a school or work lunch may include (in a hot insulated food container) stews, boiled meat balls or patties, any leftovers from a hot meal, or rolled pancakes. Subsequent stages may contain any of the above or avocado sticks; previously cooked, cold chicken chunks rolled into big lettuce pieces to form a wrap; cold baked or grilled chicken; eggs (boiled, scrambled, or omelette) in a hot- or cold-insulated food container; baby carrots; "fries" made of thinly cut butternut squash, acorn squash, onions, celery, or carrots; patties or balls made of nuts; salad enhanced with nuts, veggies, homemade dressing, and/or cubed cheese; fruit; a mash of tuna, pickles, and celery; cold bacon; grass-fed beef hotdog wieners in nut flour wraps; homemade sliced lunch meat; dehydrated fruit; apple slices dehydrated with cinnamon and dipped in nut butter; or homemade beef jerky.

My son's school snack and lunch typically includes a 500 mL (2 cups) portion of that morning's breakfast (e.g., stew, soup, beef risotto, scrambled eggs, or cooked fish) still hot and transported in a heat-insulated food container, plus a separate container of sliced cheese or pepperoni with veggies (e.g., tomato, cucumber, or carrots). In a pinch, I dump canned tuna or salmon into a cold-insulated food container. Once in a blue moon, I include in his lunch a coconut flour biscuit. His school does not allow nuts, so I reserve our limited nut products for an after-school snack. If your child's daycare centre or school does not allow food to be brought from home, explain your child's unique circumstances to the administrators and, if necessary, bring a note from your health care practitioner stating that this diet is medically necessary (see this Guide's section *Special Considerations: Communicating with Others*). If these steps do not bring results, you might consider finding a new child care centre or school, or even homelearning.

Almost anything you take to school or work now, you can take on GAPS— the only difference is you need to make it yourself, out of permitted ingredients. Again, any conventional recipe can be transposed into a GAPS dish, and you can find GAPS-friendly recipes for wraps, sandwich bread, etc., in cookbooks and online. To locate menu plans specific to any point during Intro or beyond, see this Guide's *Recipes: More Essentials–More Recipes for Intro and Beyond* section.

Supper

For my son and me, this meal has the most variety. It's determined by what we have eaten already that day, our remaining appetite, how much energy I have to prepare food, and so on. Generally, I don't start prepping a convoluted meal at the end of a long day. Thus, supper might be two plums each with a glass of kefir, or it might be "spaghetti" (spiralized zucchini) under a mound of tomato-veggie sauce with or without ground beef or meatballs, or any other dish.

Full-Time Work or School

When you will be away from home for many hours, one of the simplest things to do is to set a soup or stew to simmer while you shower and dress in the morning, have the soup or stew (or eggs or another quick meal) for breakfast, and take your hot food with you in insulated food containers for lunch and snacks.

While taking a short walking break from reworking this Guide, I came upon a man who had been working very hard in the hot weather to replace a fence near my home. I did a double-take when I realized this construction worker was preparing a massive, GAPS-friendly lunch on the tailgate of his pickup truck! He was cooking huge steaks on a compact, propane-powered barbeque grill. Although we did not speak the same language, we had a happy moment celebrating his ingenuity together!

Some people set up a slow-cooker first thing in the morning, and come home to their supper already made. Some support list members who are students have been able to arrange for disability accommodations (i.e., a room with cooking facilities).

Other list members create a week's worth of dishes on the weekend (if without kitchen facilities, then at a friend's house), freeze some, and then enjoy them all week. A community kitchen is a non-profit program that helps individuals connect with others of similar dietary needs and, together, access a commercial kitchen in order to make multiple meals in a short time and at reduced cost. Invite folks in your area with gut dysbiosis to join you in forming one.

Travel

Many GAPSters travel for pleasure, work, or even in regular evacuation from severe weather systems! Some things list members suggest include:

- Travelling by car so you can bring coolers or even plug in a tiny fridge
- Bringing insulated food containers onto the bus and/or ferry
- Distracting children with fun and books rather than with food
- Bringing a portable barbeque grill
- Using a traveller's hostel or a motel room with a kitchenette (make a pot of stew, fill a day's worth of insulated food containers, and head out)
- Shopping for food as soon as you arrive at your destination
- Requesting a note from your doctor indicating that you require a medical diet. This may allow you to bring broths and other staples onto a plane and/or across borders.

Using an Insulated Food Container

With an insulated food container, all GAPS food is portable and the need for microwave use is eliminated. For our family of two, I own four insulated food containers by Thermos®. These make our lives much easier. During Intro, we carry the soups in multiple containers. Outside of early Intro, my son's school lunch fills one insulated food container and his snack or cold lunch additions (e.g., cheese and cucumber slices) travel alongside in a separate, non-insulated container. I prefer a wide-mouth insulated food container with no frills. These are easy to fill, easy to eat from, and easy to wash. Ours have held up for four years of almost daily use so far.

The key to using an insulated food container is preconditioning it (preparing it) for hot or cold food. Depending on the temperature you want the food served at, fill the container with either very hot or very cold tap water, put the lid on, let it sit for five to ten minutes, then dump the water out. Add hot food to a heat-conditioned food container, or cold food to a cold-conditioned one. Fill the insulated food container to the top. Screw the lid on. You're set! The fuller the insulated food container, the longer the food will retain its preferred temperature (this can be critical for food safety); insulated food containers that are only partially full will lose their temperature more quickly. Opening the lid throughout the day will also result in temperature losses; try to use all the food in one sitting.

Food Details

Although a list of GAPS-friendly foods is offered below, there is more to the food aspect of the program than what we eat. Different foods are suitable for different points in our healing, and how a food is prepared is often also relevant. While using the list as a quick reference point, please also refer regularly to the following food notes.

Primary foods: Depending on your personal tolerances, the following foods should form the bulk of your diet: fats, marrow, and soft tissue from the insides of animals, fresh or frozen meats and organ meats, eggs, fish, shellfish, fresh vegetables, garlic, and olive oil. Raw vegetables (either whole or juiced), fats, approximately 250 mL (1 cup) of broth, and fermented food should be included with every meal. Fruits should be eaten away from other foods.

Forms of foods: Any permitted food can be consumed in any form as long as the given form is tolerated. Thus, any of the listed foods may be processed at home into a milk, juice, oil, or butter, or dried, roasted, salted, or fermented. For example, almonds are listed so pure almond milk and almond oil—if tolerated—are fine; coconut is listed so coconut flour and coconut water kefir are fine. Note that tolerance can be impacted by the form ingested. For example, even if whole coconut (which includes its fat and liquid) is well tolerated, coconut flour (highly concentrated in fibre) may not be. Whole carrots, which contain fibre to slow their digestion, may be tolerated long before a cup of carrot juice is, as this is very high in sugars and absorbed quickly into the body. Generally speaking, the more extracted from its source or otherwise processed an item is (e.g., coconut sugar crystals or commercial stevia powder), the more challenging it will be for the body to tolerate it. As much as possible, aim for whole forms of foods. Finally, as detailed subsequently, commercial versions of any product may contain other non-GAPS ingredients, in which case processing at home is the way to go.

Commercially processed: Not all countries require food processors to list all of the ingredients in packaged foods. When an additive makes up a small percentage of the "product" and does not have to be listed, it may still prove hard on your body. Also, the chemicals used in packaging—those in meat wrapping papers, or bisphenol A (BPA) in the lining of many cans, for example—may cause symptoms, whether immediate or delayed, in some people. It is always safest to use foods in their whole form and process them yourself. If you decide to use a commercially processed food, be sure to use only those without any non-GAPS ingredients included. I encourage you to write to the company and ask what other items were used in the food's processing or included in the packaging.

Tolerances: Not all GAPS foods will be tolerated by all people, especially early on. Legumes and flours tend to be the most commonly challenging and may need to be delayed for some time. For many people, proper preparation (e.g., fermenting beans and soaking nuts and seeds) is key. However, some healing time may be required before even a properly prepared food becomes a tolerated one. Fruits, sweet vegetables (e.g., carrots, beets, and orange squashes), and honey also trigger challenges for some people. Regarding tolerance, the Intro progression—and a methodical approach in general—are very helpful. These are detailed throughout this Guide.

Stages: As mentioned earlier, not all GAPS-recommended foods are immediately digestible. For example, raw produce is very healthy, but may be very hard on a compromised system. After an appropriate transition to the program, as detailed in this Guide, the Intro progression will provide maximum—and most efficient—healing. In Intro, you will start with the most digestible items, such as well-cooked, non-fibrous vegetables in meat broth. As the gut begins to heal and rebuild, in most people raw produce will be successfully introduced about four weeks into Intro.

Meats/fish: Most meats/fish (e.g., beef, goose, duck, chicken, buffalo, halibut, sole, salmon, sardines, and most other meats and fish) are recommended. These should be purchased either fresh or frozen, and otherwise not commercially processed (i.e., salted or dried). An exception is fish canned in water or in its own juice, which is fine. Preferably, meats should be wild or grass-fed, but if your body tolerates the various foods and antibiotics fed to some animals, any source is acceptable. In her FAQ document, Dr. Campbell-McBride recommends that tuna (although it is in the list of permitted foods) and other large carnivorous fish such as shark should be avoided if possible.

Dairy: For those who can tolerate it, the GAPS program recommends ghee or butter as well as dairy that has been fermented sufficiently to reduce lactose. If you are keen on a cheese which is not listed, check with the manufacturer about its age and lactose level. For more information on dairy in GAPS, see this Guide's section *Food Issues: Dairy*.

Beans: Beans (except string beans), lentils, and split peas should be fermented before further preparation. Please see the *Recipes: Ferments* section of this Guide.

Seeds and nuts: Buy nuts in their original state, either shelled or unshelled. Nuts that are commercially oiled or commercially roasted are not to be used. Feel free to process them at home, though, in any way that you like. Dr. Campbell-McBride recommends that sunflower, pumpkin, and sesame seeds be properly soaked for 12 hours. She notes that some bodies demand that nuts be soaked, too. Please see detailed instructions in the *Recipes: More Essentials* section of this Guide.

Coconut flour: After sufficient healing, this very fibrous food can be used cautiously and in moderation.

Fruits: If tolerated at all, fruits should be eaten when truly ripe. Generally, this means they should be falling off a local plant. A banana must be ripened enough to display dark speckles across it. Ideally, fruits are eaten on their own, at least 30 minutes before, or two to three hours after, meals containing other foods. Also, be aware that commercially dried fruits often include additives. As with all foods, whole and unprocessed fruits are best.

Bone broth: Because some people can react to this, I recommend approaching bone broth (as opposed to meat broth) as an advanced food, testing it any time after completing Intro.

What to Include

The following foods are those generally recommended for GAPS. Any food on the list that is not tolerated by a given individual should be omitted from one's personal program (if an intolerance requires you to exclude a food, be sure to see the *Food Issues: Food Sensitivities/Allergies* section of this Guide, and to retest the food regularly). Again, if possible, each food should be purchased in its whole state and then processed at home. Commercially processed foods should be limited as much as possible, with the exceptions of fish canned in water or its own juice, olives, tomato purée or tomato juice, butter, oils, cheese, and so on. Also limit canned foods as much as possible to avoid chemicals such as BPA.

Almonds, including almond butter and oil
Apples
Apricots, fresh or dried
Artichoke, French
Asiago cheese
Asparagus
Aubergine/eggplant
Avocados, including avocado oil

Bananas, ripe with brown spots on the peel
Beans, dried white (navy), haricot, string beans, lima beans, properly prepared
Beef, fresh or frozen
Beets or beetroot
Berries, all kinds
Black, white and red pepper (ground and pepper corns)

Black radish
Blue cheese
Bok choy
Brazil nuts
Brick cheese
Brie cheese
Broccoli
Brussels sprouts
Butter
Cabbage
Camembert cheese
Canned fish, in oil or water only
Capers
Carrots
Cashew nuts, fresh only
Cauliflower
Cayenne pepper
Celeriac
Celery
Cellulose in supplements
Cheddar cheese
Cherimoya/custard apple/sharifa
Cherries
Chicken, fresh or frozen
Cinnamon
Citric acid
Coconut, fresh or dried (shredded)
    without any additives
Coconut milk
Coconut oil
Coffee, weak and freshly made (not
    instant)
Collard greens
Colby cheese
Courgette/zucchini
Coriander, fresh or dried
Cucumber
Dates, fresh or dried without any additives
Dill, fresh or dried
Duck, fresh or frozen
Edam cheese
Eggplant/aubergine
Eggs, fresh
Filberts
Fish, fresh or frozen, canned in oil or its
    juice
Game, fresh or frozen
Garlic
Ghee, homemade
Gin, occasionally

Ginger root, fresh
Goose, fresh or frozen
Gorgonzola cheese
Gouda cheese
Grapefruit
Grapes
Haricot beans, properly prepared
Havarti cheese
Hazelnuts
Herbal teas
Herbs, fresh or dried without additives
Honey, preferably raw
Juices freshly pressed from permitted fruit
    and vegetables
Kale
Kefir (per SCD or GAPS recipes)
Kiwi fruit
Kumquats
Lamb, fresh or frozen
Lemons
Lentils, properly prepared
Lettuce, all kinds
Lima beans, dried and fresh (properly
    prepared)
Limburger cheese
Limes
Mangoes
Meats, fresh or frozen, including insects
Melons
Monterey Jack cheese
Muenster cheese
Mushrooms
Mustard seeds, pure powder and gourmet
    types
Nectarines
Nut flour or ground nuts (usually ground
    blanched almonds)
Nutmeg
Nuts, freshly shelled, not commercially
    roasted, salted, or coated
Olive oil, cold-pressed
Olives
Onions
Oranges
Papayas
Parmesan cheese
Parsley
Peaches
Peanut butter, without additives
Peanuts, fresh or roasted in their shells

Pears

Peas, dried split (properly prepared) and fresh green

Pecans

Peppers (green, yellow, red, and orange)

Pheasant, fresh or frozen

Pickles, without sugar or any other non-allowed ingredients

Pigeon, fresh or frozen

Pineapples, fresh

Pork, fresh or frozen

Port-du-Salut cheese

Poultry, fresh or frozen

Prunes, dried without any additives or in their own juice

Pumpkin

Quail, fresh or frozen

Raisins

Rhubarb

Roquefort cheese

Romano cheese

Satsumas

Scotch, occasionally

Seaweed fresh or dried, once Intro is completed

Shellfish, fresh or frozen

Spices, single and pure without any additives

Spinach

Squash (summer and winter)

Stilton cheese

String beans

Swedes

Swiss cheese

Tangerines

Tea, weak, freshly made (not instant)

Tomato purée, without additives (except salt)

Tomato juice, without additives (except salt)

Tomatoes

Turkey, fresh or frozen

Turnips

Ugli fruit

Uncreamed cottage cheese ("dry curd")

Vinegar (cider or white)

Vodka, very occasionally

Walnuts

Watercress

White navy beans, properly prepared

Whey (per SCD or GAPS recipes only)

Wine, dry (red or white)

Yogurt (per SCD or GAPS recipes)

Zucchini (courgette)

Additional Foods

Generally speaking, we would avoid any food not listed in the *What to Include* section. However, in her FAQ document (see *Using this Guide*), Dr. Campbell-McBride notes that upon sufficient healing of obvious digestive issues, a number of other foods may be included in Full GAPS, as personal tolerance allows. These include, but are not limited to: *Aloe vera*; bee pollen; chlorophyll; pure cocoa; colostrum; homemade kombucha; sea plants, such as dulse and seaweed; small amounts of fresh or home-dried stevia herb; nettles (not during pregnancy); all other herbs (initially in extracts and teas and eventually eaten in their fibrous whole); and sprouted legumes. For additional or subsequent updates as to which foods are encouraged within the dietary aspect of GAPS, every month review Dr. Campbell-McBride's FAQ document. Use the "search" or "find" function to locate all references in the document to the food under consideration (e.g., different places in the FAQ document may offer varying information per medical condition).

Any food not listed in the *What to Include* section, I would test only after having completed a full round of Intro followed by a minimum of three to six months of Full GAPS without any symptoms, whether digestive, cognitive, mood, or other. The only exception I would make is if a specific food is indicated in Dr. Campbell-McBride's FAQ document to help resolve a persistent symptom. If upon consideration an additional food seems to be a possible fit for your body, test it and watch for any effects. If your body accepts the additional food, jot it down alongside the *What to Include* list.

With respect to baking soda (bicarbonate of soda), in the November 2010 edition of her book, Dr. Campbell-McBride lists pure bicarbonate of soda as an exception to the avoid list. However, in her FAQ document, Dr. Campbell-McBride reiterates that bicarbonate of soda is not to be used as an ingredient in food recipes, due to its potential to reduce desired stomach acid. (In the same document, Dr. Campbell-McBride notes that it may, however, be used internally or externally as a remedy for specific issues, such as *Candida* overgrowth and reflux.) Many people are concerned their baking will not turn out well without the use of baking soda. GAPSters find that most baking recipes work fine without baking soda. Also, baking recipes developed specifically for GAPS will naturally exclude baking soda and have excellent results without it. Some GAPSters have tested using baking soda and report that a small amount in the occasional recipe is tolerated by them.

Regarding flax, Dr. Campbell-McBride has discouraged its use in some references. However, in May 2012, she stated in her FAQ document that flax oil (if combined with other oils) and flax seeds are allowed upon sufficient digestive healing.

Supplements, vitamins, and minerals can be added after several months of healing—including a round of Intro—if the body indicates a need for more support. Please see details in the *Supplementation: Other Supplements* section of this Guide.

What to Avoid

Of course it is not possible for Dr. Campbell-McBride to categorize every single food under the sun. Ideally, you will avoid any food not yet mentioned in the list of recommended foods, or in a list of exceptions, or in the most recent version of Dr. Campbell-McBride's FAQ document.

Despite the relative clarity of this statement, I regularly receive enquiries along the following lines: "Can I eat [potatoes, maple syrup, molasses, commercial stevia, etc.]?" Again, any food not mentioned in the list of recommended foods, in the references to advanced foods or exceptions (as noted in this Guide or elsewhere), or in Dr. Campbell-McBride's FAQ document should not be ingested.

Although the above answers the question of commercial stevia powder, this particular query comes up so often, by people who have such a strong desire to use this item, it deserves its own notation. In general, the only sweeteners permitted on GAPS are honey and fruit (fresh or dried). Dr. Campbell-McBride does not generally support the use of stevia. An exception she makes is for small amounts of fresh or home-dried stevia (which would fit under the general category of herbs). Some people who are very sensitive to both honey and fruit have used commercial stevia with their "otherwise GAPS" program. To my knowledge, they report no adverse side effects, and express that this source of sweetness allows them to otherwise stick with the program. Ideally, one will use just fruit and honey as sweeteners, but when fruit and honey are truly an issue, the question of whether to use commercial stevia or not will need to be a discussion between you and your health practitioner (as with all points in this Guide).

Are you are wondering about other items or about why a given food is on the avoid list? Please see the *Special Considerations: Need for Proof* section in this Guide. Referenced there are options for completing more extensive research on any given item or aspect of the program.

When you have assessed yourself as having achieved sufficient healing, it will be your prerogative to test any food not explicitly recommended for GAPS. However, do be aware that the effects of some foods may be slow and/or cumulative. Again, it is recommended to commit a minimum of 18–24 months to strict GAPS before moving on to foods or diets not explicitly recommended by Dr. Campbell-McBride.

Post-GAPS

After having completed your full healing program, which for most people requires a minimum of 18–24 months, and you have been free of symptoms for at least six months, you can begin to test additional foods, including properly prepared grains. Ideally, you will first test new potatoes (if GAPS nightshades such as tomatoes and eggplant have been well tolerated) or fermented, gluten-free grains (e.g., fermented buckwheat, fermented millet, and fermented quinoa). If these are well tolerated, homemade sourdough can be tested. Once their gut is fully healed, many people experience another surge in health after adding these nutrient-dense, properly prepared starches as a minor adjunct (i.e., an enhancement) to their otherwise GAPS menu. At this stage in the journey, most bodies welcome these and utilize them well.

After completing GAPS, most people find they are able to tolerate any food. However, ingesting poor quality foods frequently or in significant amounts—especially when this results in a low volume of nutrient-dense foods being ingested—will likely cause health issues to return. Through continued experimentation—and consultation as needed—you will determine the optimal long-term diet for you.

Through the post-GAPS phase of additional trial and error, a few people find they cannot tolerate anything outside of the basic GAPS protocol, experiencing their optimal health only by staying with the program permanently. This is more likely to be true for adults with severe issues, such as schizophrenia, who started GAPS relatively late in life.

For many who have required GAPS to heal intense health issues, the ideal post-GAPS diet might be that advocated by The Weston A. Price Foundation, a paleolithic one, a continuation of Full GAPS, or a "mostly GAPS" diet with the occasional or regular ingestion of non-GAPS food. The latter is what my son and I have done.

CHAPTER 3

DETOXIFICATION

A damaged gut produces a lot of toxins. Items we use every day, as well as elements in our general environment, may also be toxic. As Dr. Campbell-McBride notes, the human body has a "detoxification system" that is responsible for the elimination of internal and environmental toxins. If this system is overloaded and cannot process the volume of toxins present, the toxic substances are stored in various tissues of one's body (e.g., skin, joints, and muscles). This causes symptoms. Although the diet and supplements will go far to reduce the overall toxic load, they cannot in themselves relieve the body of years of accumulated muck. Additional steps are needed. Detox supports, such as home-pressed juices, supplemented baths, and daily bowel movements, can help remove the existing load as well as any unpreventable new burdens. Conscious lifestyle choices can limit any further unnecessary exposures.

Within the context of GAPS, "detoxifying" or "detoxing" refers to the removal of toxins from one's body. The body does this naturally, every day. To speed healing, we can support this process in several ways. Every positive choice can help, and for some people even a single change (e.g., filtering chlorine from their bathing water or eliminating detergents from their body care product line) can make all the difference. I continue to believe that what we put directly into our mouths is the most critical piece. Thus, when financial constraints demand that a choice be made, I prefer to see people focus their money on whole, preferably organic, foods rather than on new shower heads or special cookware.

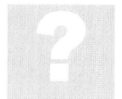

"WHEN I DID AN ELIMINATION DIET BEFORE, I GOT HORRIBLY SICK. I CAN'T BEAR TO GET SICK LIKE THAT AGAIN."

The sickness was likely intense "die-off." When pathogenic microbes die off, they release toxins. When the toxins are produced faster than your body can process/remove them, you experience die-off symptoms. Each round is temporary, usually lasting 3–4 days, but possibly up to several weeks. If planned and managed, symptoms of intense die-off can be reduced or, in some cases, prevented altogether. To some degree, you're in charge. Planning a gentle approach will be worth it because it will be much more comfortable and will help you hang in for the long haul.

Diet's Role in Detox

In several ways, the diet aspect of GAPS vastly reduces the amount of toxins in our bodies. Its focus on unprocessed, nutrient-dense food eliminates artificial chemicals, dyes, and those foods (e.g., soy) that may trigger hormone imbalances. Further, in using only foods that are quickly digested and do not remain in the gut to feed an imbalance of microbes, the amount of toxins that would otherwise be generated internally is reduced. Finally, the diet's live enzymes, probiotics, phenols, and other elements offer "cleaning services" to the body, helping to eliminate built-up toxins. In all of these ways, the diet is key to reducing toxins in the body!

Bowel Movements

Daily release of stool is a critical component to the detoxification aspect of the GAPS healing protocol. Bowel movements become such a point of concern for people doing GAPS that it is worth delving into the details.

In the first months of healing, stool changes are very common. Regardless of how well you adhere to the program, in the early stages your stool may be black, white, tarry, mucousy, loose, liquid, foul-smelling, floating, sinking, balled, coiled, large, small, and so on. It may contain visible fats or undigested vegetables. Bowel movements may occur just once every few days (in which case intervention must be implemented), once a day, or several times per day. As long as a person is having at least one bowel movement per day, this is sufficient.

Stool changes are indicative of changes in the body overall. Again, regardless of what you eat, drink, or bathe in, periods of deep healing will bring an array of stool types. Overall, we can recognize this as a transient issue and ignore the details. As healing progresses, the stool will become more consistent. After some weeks or months on the program, it will present more consistently as brown, formed as either blobs or a length, and not be overly offensive in scent. In the meantime, allow for stool changes and focus more on the other changes in terms of progressing through the program (e.g., behaviour, emotion, and skin).

Five issues that may require special attention are: suspected food intolerances, severe intestinal issues (e.g., Crohn's disease, irritable bowel syndrome, or ulcerative colitis), red colour associated with the bowels or stool, true diarrhea, and constipation. Each of these is explored in the pages that follow.

Suspected Food Intolerances and Stool

If you suspect a specific food of triggering troublesome stool (e.g., constipation, loose stools, or undigested food), remove the food for two weeks, then reintroduce it. If the trigger is confirmed, remove that food for several more weeks or longer while further healing takes place, and then retest it. For more details on this approach, read the *Food Issues: Testing for Food Sensitivities* section of this Guide.

Severe Intestinal Issues

Please see the notes in a subsequent section of this Guide, *Health Issues: Severe Intestinal Issues,* and the *Detoxification: Bowel Movements–Diarrhea* section, if applicable.

Red Colour

Sometimes the colour red associated with stool is benign; sometimes it's not. Red stool (or urine) can result from eating red food, such as beets, in which case the colour is not a concern. Sometimes pushing out a large, constipated stool can cause irritation—to the point of light bleeding—at the end of the canal, resulting in small amounts of blood attached to the stool or visible in the toilet or on the toilet paper. A small tear should heal on its own, and resolving constipation will prevent this issue in the future. Bleeding from anywhere inside the bowels is often resolved (either quickly or eventually) through GAPS, but in the meantime, this symptom should be cared for by a health practitioner.

Diarrhea

In the early stages of healing, or during a healing crisis at any other point during the program, many people will experience one to three mushy, loose, or liquid stools in a day. This "acute release" can be part of healing. In supporting peers through the GAPS protocol, I define "true diarrhea" as *more than three very loose or liquid stools that also cause one to race to the bathroom.* Although an occasional loose stool may not require any specific attention, true diarrhea can result in dehydration very quickly and must be addressed. True diarrhea that lasts days or weeks can also result in other types of malnourishment and must be addressed more aggressively, under the direction of a health practitioner.

At the onset of any degree of diarrhea, try the following:

• Incorporate an electrolyte drink to maintain critical hydration and mineral levels.

• Stop vegetables. Once you have been clear of true diarrhea for at least three days, restart them using only the parts that are non-fibrous, do not include peels or seeds, and cook them well. For example, use cauliflower or broccoli florets, but not the stems or stalks; use zucchini, but not the seeded core. Carrots and mushrooms are also good choices.

• If you started a probiotic source (e.g., yogurt, kefir, or a capsule) a short time before the diarrhea began, this may have been the trigger (especially if the probiotic was started at a relatively high dose, such as half a capsule). Stop the probiotic altogether. When the diarrhea resolves, start your probiotic at a beginning dose, working up very slowly from there (see this Guide's section *Supplementation: Probiotics*).

- If you are not yet taking a probiotic source, one might help. Start one now, beginning with a tiny amount and working up very slowly (see this Guide's section *Supplementation: Probiotics*).

- If using dairy, remove high-fat dairy (e.g., ghee, butter, and sour cream) and incorporate high-protein dairy (e.g., whey, yogurt, and kefir).

- Consider a course of *Saccharomyces boulardii* (*S. boulardii*), a friendly yeast that often resolves diarrhea (see the *Progressing Further* section of this Guide).

If these do not remedy the issue sufficiently, or if the diarrhea is severe and immediate relief is required, consider the temporary use of *Aloe vera* juice. Even one or two doses, at the amount recommended by the manufacturer, can provide emergency relief, preventing further issues like dehydration or soreness, and allowing one to move forward with the healing progression. If using *Aloe vera* juice as an emergency remedy, be sure to apply the previous tips for this condition as well.

Constipation

Are your movements not happening daily? Are they slow, painful, or overly large? Are they like small stones rather than gentle blobs or an easy length? Many people coming to GAPS have struggled for years with constipation. Others become constipated temporarily on the GAPS Intro. Some are certain this is due to the reduction in fibre in early Intro, but what we actually observe is that constipation returns with each round of die-off in many people, regardless of how much fibre has been incorporated into the diet (think of breast-fed infants who take in no fibre, yet are not constipated unless unwell).

In her book, *Gut and Psychology Syndrome*, Dr. Campbell-McBride indicates that daily bowel movements are crucial to health recovery and maintenance. She notes that the diet soon resolves constipation in most people. In the meantime, she generally recommends no supplemental laxatives and strongly supports the use of enemas any time 36 hours have passed without a bowel movement. For detailed information on enemas, please see the relevant section of this Guide.

Other approaches that have worked for people on our support list, or which are suggested in Dr. Campbell-McBride's FAQ document, are presented below. My recommendation is to try each one in turn, starting with whichever feels most accessible to you and testing it for four to seven days before moving on to a new remedy. During Intro, try to use a stage-friendly remedy, but if none of those works, feel free to use any other one. Any supplement listed below should be taken as directed by its manufacturer or by your health care practitioner.

Long-Term Solutions

The GAPS program is the primary long-term solution for constipation. Do the program patiently, ultimately achieving a gut balanced in flora and able to support all of the body's necessary processes. Incorporate all aspects of the program such as Intro, Full GAPS, detoxification, and supplementation. In addition to these, the following tweaks may help you find your body's optimal program.

- For some people, starting a homemade or commercial probiotic will trigger constipation. This is likely due to die-off. For others, however, a sufficient probiotic count is what will finally regulate movements. To limit the possibility of die-off triggering constipation, ensure probiotics are properly introduced and then increase them slowly. See this Guide's section *Supplementation: Probiotics*.

- Regardless of constipation, continue moving forward in the Intro progression. The healing that occurs through building a nutrient-dense diet may resolve the issue. Also, sometimes a specific food will prove helpful to moving the bowels. In one person, this may be butternut squash; in another, it may be nut butter or fermented vegetables. As in all aspects of GAPS, moving forward can be critical to resolving issues.

- Increase fats from the inside of animals and gelatinous meats.

- Increase cooked vegetables (especially beets). Although GAPS relies on bacteria, not fibre, to produce bowel movements, for some people vegetables will help move the bowels. At various times, cooked and/or raw vegetables may comprise up to 80% of your GAPS diet.

- Eliminate problematic foods. See the section *Food Issues: Food Sensitivities/Allergies* in this Guide. If the cooked beets suggested previously do not resolve the constipation, Dr. Campbell-McBride suggests that those with persistent constipation remove all sweet vegetables (e.g., carrots, beets, and orange squash) from their diet temporarily.

- If including dairy, incorporate high-fat dairy (especially sour cream, but also ghee and butter).

- Remove high-protein dairy (e.g., whey, yogurt, kefir, and cheese).

- Reduce muscle meats.

- At least 20 minutes before breakfast, drink the following mixture: high-magnesium juiced produce (e.g., greens, beets, cabbage, carrots, celery, apples, and oranges) with raw egg and sour cream whisked in. If dairy-free, start your day with the freshly pressed juice of oranges or grapefruits.

- Add 15 mL (1 tablespoon) of apple cider vinegar to 250 mL (1 cup) of room temperature water. Sip this throughout the day. Additionally, take a full cup of this mixture 15 minutes before a meal.

- Any source of fat (e.g., broth, GAPS' bottled oils, or olive oil) may help produce bowel movements. Add fat to everything. For one child on our support list, 5 mL (1 teaspoon) of lemon-flavoured liquid Carlson's cod liver oil taken directly from a spoon and chased with some water just before bed eliminated the extreme pain he'd previously experienced with bowel movements and resolved the need for enemas.

- *S. boulardii* (see the *Progressing Further* section of this Guide). Often used to resolve diarrhea, this friendly yeast also resolves constipation for some.

- Physical movement, such as stretching, twisting, walking, yoga, or gentle dance, can help produce regular bowel movements.

Interim Remedies

The following remedies can be applied as needed—even daily for a time, if required. However, we want to rely primarily on rebuilding the gut's natural balance so that the body can move the bowels on its own. Although the following can be used to help remove toxins from the body and relieve discomfort, be sure to continue applying all aspects of the GAPS program, as well as any of the tips presented previously.

- Enema (detailed in the subsequent *Enemas* section).

- Epsom salt baths.

- At the beginning of each meal, take betaine hydrochloride (HCL) with pepsin in the ratio presented in this Guide's *Supplementation* section. For resolving constipation, an adult may require one to two capsules.

- Supplement with spirulina, blue-green algae, chlorella, or dunaliella, if tolerated (and other extreme digestive issues do not contraindicate).

- Address poor fat digestion. Review the information in this Guide under *Health Issues: Fat Malabsorption.*

- Add an oral magnesium supplement. Dr. Campbell-McBride recommends amino acid chelates of magnesium—daily for as long as is required—or magnesium oxide occasionally. Many GAPSters initially use a supplement such as Magnesium Citrate Powder by Natural Calm Canada (www.naturalcalm.ca) to bowel tolerance (i.e., increasing the dose until stools are loose, then continuing to use the dose immediately previous to that one). As your range of food increases, you will be able to access increasing amounts of magnesium—with the same effects—through GAPS foods and juices.

- Take vitamin C to bowel tolerance (i.e., increasing the dose until stools are loose, then continuing to use the dose immediately previous to that one). As your range of food increases, you will be able to access increasing amounts of vitamin C—with the same effects—through GAPS foods and juices.

- Eat cooked fruits, especially apples, plums, or prunes (adding soaked nuts, such as walnuts, may also help), preferably first thing in the morning, with nothing else until 10 AM or so. Use approximately 125–250 mL (½–1 cup). If still no movement after four to six hours, have another dose.

- For occasional use, an application of castor oil on the belly, covered with a hot towel and hot water bottle can be helpful. Alternatively, castor oil can be taken orally (note that castor oil is contraindicated during pregnancy).

- Some people have reported good results with professional colonics, preferring them to a do-it-yourself enema.

- Use rewards with children. Children who seem constipated may suddenly be able to move their bowels after a promise of a favourite food or activity (e.g., story, outing, or video). Some children with a history of constipation have become fearful of bowel movements. Other children are loath to interrupt play for such a boring activity. A reward may make a bowel movement "worth it." With my son, ensuring regular bowel movements early in healing required that I say, "Yes, you can play (or watch a movie or have a snack)…right after you poop!" Granted, sometimes his body had nothing to release at that point and he was off the hook, but frequently there was and he simply wouldn't attend to this need unless a favourite activity was delayed for it.

- Allow your body a regular time for a bowel movement. Don't override this appointment with anything else—your colon is counting on you! For most people, first thing in the morning or right after breakfast works best.

- When sitting on the toilet, draw your knees up toward your chest (put a stool or flipped-over wastepaper basket on the floor and rest your feet on that).

This puts your body in a position more amenable to moving stool out. Alternatively, while sitting on the toilet, gently and repeatedly twist the upper half of your body as far to the left and as far to the right as you can.

- Gently massage the abdomen. It is particularly helpful to massage in the direction in which stool transits through the colon.
- On occasion, a glycerin suppository for a child is fine.

Enemas

The following information is largely collated from the book *Gut and Psychology Syndrome* (9th edition) by Dr. Campbell-McBride with notes by GAPS community member Sarah Lascano.

As with all health approaches (e.g., supplementation, changes to diet, and physical procedures), enemas do carry a risk. The right supplies and approach for a given age can be critical. With GAPS, enemas may be used occasionally or daily to relieve the bowels or to release a toxic overload. Some people have reported fast and dramatic changes in skin condition, mood, behaviour, digestion, and more with the use of an enema.

For specific symptoms, Dr. Campbell-McBride also recommends enemas incorporating garlic, bicarbonate of soda, coffee, chamomile tea, or *Aloe vera*. For the circumstances in which to use these, plus recipes and procedures for each, please see Dr. Campbell-McBride's FAQ document.

Keep a child happy throughout the process with books, conversation, and so on. Ensure the experience is positive and pleasant. Many people assume their child will resist and hate an enema. Some children have indeed found the process upsetting and have subsequently relied on other options to move the bowels. However, a number of families have reported that their children were not upset by the process, and that the children actually responded to a completed enema by laughing, singing, and playing. The children's positive associations with the procedure and results are such that every time they feel overwhelmed by symptoms, they request another!

If an enema has been used daily for several weeks or months, and the Full GAPS diet plus the other tips for moving the bowels have been incorporated in the meantime, please see Dr. Campbell-McBride's FAQ document for instructions on transitioning from daily enemas.

Supplies

Enema kits can be found in many drug stores and online. Simply do an Internet search for "enema kit" and many options, including those described next, will come up. Essentially, an enema requires a container for fluid, a tube or hose to transport the fluid, and a nozzle for insertion into the anus. Each piece of reusable equipment must be easy to clean thoroughly.

A standard enema bag has several advantages: it works well, you can fill it yourself, it holds plenty of water for an adult, and it is available in many drug stores. A challenge with these is that you cannot see how much water is moving into the body (relevant when administering to a child), the tip isn't as comfortable as some, the tip can unscrew frequently, and the hose can kink (though it is also easily straightened). A stainless steel bucket designed for enemas has many of the same pros and cons, with some kits being completely latex-free. A see-through bag allows you to observe how much fluid is going in.

While not as thorough, a disposable Fleet enema will work in a pinch and is relatively convenient and comfortable. Empty it of its commercial solution and refill it with your own. The commercial solutions usually rely on a chemical irritant, so when using the emptied container with water-plus-probiotic, more volume is needed. One list member said, "For my [three-year-old] son, I needed up to three to four of the pediatric ones filled with water."

For Young Children

Three excellent options for children include the disposable Fleet enema as described previously, a bulb syringe enema, or a regular enema kit with a smaller, softer, more flexible nozzle. To locate the latter, do an Internet search for a phrase such as "flex-tip enema nozzle junior."

! **IMPORTANT**

Do not use an enema if rectal bleeding is present.

Administering a Full Enema

1. Buy the enema kit of your choice and all other supplies (e.g., *Aloe vera* gel and child-friendly tip) listed in these steps.
2. If the kit contains a commercial solution, pour it out.
3. Boil 2 litres (8 cups) of filtered or bottled water.
4. Cool it down to a temperature that will be safe and comfortable internally (e.g., 20°C–40°C).
5. Assemble the enema kit.
6. Hang the enema bucket 1 metre (3 feet) above where you will be lying down.
7. Fill the enema bag with clean water (but not the water you boiled).
8. Open the enema kit's tap and let all the water flush through.

9. Close the kit's tap.
10. Fill the enema bag with the boiled and cooled water.
11. Let some of the water flush through to clean out any impurities.
12. Close the tap.
13. Fill the bag with the remaining warm water. Add a probiotic to the bag of water. Use one with predominantly *Bifidobacterium* in it. The enema water will need to contain at least four to five billion viable bacterial cells. Use powder or capsule; do not use a tablet form, as this will have binders and fillers. It is acceptable, but not ideal, to use a powder or capsule containing maltodextrin or fructooligosaccharides (FOS), but note that this may cause excess gas to be produced over the subsequent day or two. Pure probiotics with no additives are best. If you cannot find a suitable probiotic, just use clean boiled water or a pure weak chamomile tea (with no ingredients besides chamomile). A few tablespoons of homemade yogurt added to the enema water can be very soothing for an inflamed or irritated rectum. Except when following directions for a different type of enema, as suggested by Dr. Campbell-McBride, do not use any products in an enema other than those listed above.
14. Set out towels to make a nice soft "bed" on the floor 1 metre (3 feet) below the enema bucket and near the toilet or potty.
15. For a child, have books, a video, or toys present for distraction.
16. Lie on your right side on the towels, in a comfortable position. For many people, this is with one's knees bent toward their chest. Lying on your right side will allow the water to travel further.
17. Apply *Aloe vera* gel or olive oil to the enema tip and anus.
18. Run the tip under warm water to warm it.
19. Insert the nozzle into the anus about 1–2 cm (approximately ½ inch) deep.
20. Partially open the tap of the enema. You want the water to flow in slowly and gently (alternatively, consider "pulsing" it in by repeatedly opening and closing the tap). For a child, 100 mL (less than ½ cup) of water may be enough initially. Eventually, a child might work up to 1 litre (4 cups). An adult can accommodate 1–2 litres. The more water you can comfortably get in, the better the cleansing.
21. Remove the nozzle from the anus. Let the water stay in for as long as is comfortable, at least five to ten minutes. While waiting, massage the belly along the route of the intestines.
22. If after ten minutes you still have not had a bowel movement, add more water.

23. Sit on the toilet for at least 10–15 minutes, allowing the bowels to empty completely. It is common, normal, and fine for that which releases from the colon to be mostly water, very minimal in water, or stool that is very small or otherwise minimal.

24. Clean the kit. Flush it through with water. Pour 20–30 mL (½–1 fluid ounce) of 3%–6% hydrogen peroxide through. With the enema tap open, hang to dry. Wash and sterilize the nozzle separately.

25. For chronic constipation, you will ideally follow the enema with a die-off relief bath, and then an abdominal rub of a quality oil (e.g., hemp, olive oil, cold-pressed sunflower oil, or castor oil—if not pregnant), and then a good night's sleep.

Die-Off Relief (Detox) Baths

The GAPS program requires a daily soak in a bath of specific solutions. Some people skip this step, not recognizing their incredible relevance and importance. Avoid this mistake! The baths actively aid healing and can bring profound relief from die-off symptoms—often immediately. During early healing, Intro, and other times of intense healing, it is important to have at least one detox bath (or foot soak) daily. Ideally, these baths are continued daily or almost daily even outside of these times.

A full body soak is ideal. However, if you do not have a tub, or if you are physically unable to get in or out of a tub (and do not own a walk-in version), soak your feet in a bucket of the same solution. The skin at all points on our body allows the transmission of key elements, and the feet seem to be an especially effective point of healing. Also, if you're not too shy, consider "borrowing" a friend's tub once a week, or asking for a friend's trained assistance in getting in and out of yours.

The optimal detox bath temperature will be different for each person and at each stage of healing. A hot detox bath may trigger more healing effects than a body is capable of processing. Start with lukewarm water and over the weeks and months of healing, work up to higher (but still safe) temperatures. Even in his fourth year of detox baths, my son uses a lukewarm temperature and still benefits. I have used very warm or hot baths right from the start, and this has been fine for me.

Follow standard safety procedures when preparing or supporting a bath for another person. Young children, seniors, and people with significant illness should be supervised for the duration of a bath, as well as assisted in and out of the tub. This can be especially important when the bath is a detoxifying one.

The bath may be at any time of the day. For one person, just before a long night's sleep might be best; for another, before the body's natural detox period ends at 10 AM is ideal. Following the bath with a nap or deep sleep provides the body with extra support.

To a full tub of water, pour any one of the following additives (use proportionately less of the chosen additive when using less than a full tub of water):

- 250 mL (1 cup) baking soda;
- 250 mL (1 cup) apple cider vinegar;
- 250 mL (1 cup) Epsom salts;
- 250 mL (1 cup) sea salts;
- 250 mL (1 cup) seaweed powder; or
- 125 mL (½ cup) baking soda and 125 mL (½ cup) Epsom salts.

Regardless of what your primary symptoms are, use a different additive each day. It is not necessary to use all five of the above additives, but do try to use at least three of the above in your rotation. Baking soda, apple cider vinegar, and Epsom salts are the most affordable and accessible to many. The rotation has various benefits, not the least of which is avoiding irritation from the salts, for example.

For constipation, an Epsom salt bath is especially helpful. For relieving detox or die-off symptoms, several have found great results mixing baking soda and Epsom salts into one bath.

Sit in the bath for at least 30 minutes. For me, I can tell when a detox bath is especially effective when the following changes occur in my body (usually about 20 minutes into the bath): my gums "sweat," my heart rate increases, I feel uncomfortable, and my feet throb. I get out when I can't stand it anymore or when the peak of these changes passes. My son displays no discomfort (perhaps because his baths are cooler) and simply plays happily in them for up to three hours.

After the bath, apply to itchy or irritated skin any of the following, as your tolerances allow: sesame oil or homemade sour cream, kefir, or yogurt (coconut oil can also be used, but may increase internal die-off).

Again, whenever possible, support your body even further by allowing it to fall into a deep sleep immediately following the soak.

A ginger bath, recommended to me by a naturopath years ago, is another option and a favourite of mine. It is detoxifying and, when taken early enough in the course of a virus, can knock a cold or flu out of one's system. Please note that in order to effectively draw the toxins out, the water for the ginger bath is supposed to be on the hot side. This bath can get uncomfortable; its effects can be similar to that of a sauna. For my son, I modify the bath to use only warm water and it still seems to help him a lot. Add 30 mL (2 tablespoons) of powdered ginger into a bath. Sit in the bath for at least 20 minutes. Close to the 20 minute mark, you may find yourself feeling intensely uncomfortable. Breathe through this; it will eventually pass. Feel free to drink cool water, or to put a cool washcloth on your forehead. With great care in case of dizziness, get out of the bath. For an enhanced experience, follow the ginger bath with a cold shower before drying off. Dry off, wrap yourself in warm blankets, and go to sleep.

Environmental Supports

House plants consume toxic gases and replace these with oxygen and other beneficial substances, so have lots of them! Also, as polluted as the outside world is, it is generally less polluted than most indoor areas, so spend as much time as possible outside, in nature, and in the sea. Open your windows. Regularly air your house out. Because they don't trap dust, mould, or chemicals, hard floors tend to support health more than carpeted ones. Over time, continue incorporating additional environmental strategies as you learn about them.

Avoiding Chemicals

Remove all chemical cleaning and personal care products (e.g., air fresheners and perfumes) from your home, car, and workspace. Do not use pesticides, carpet cleaning solutions, conventional dry cleaning services, household paints, and other common sources of chemicals. Avoid chlorinated swimming pools and other toxic water. Consider what chemicals you may be exposed to at home or at work and try to avoid those as much as possible. For example, move your work cubicle away from any source of cigarette smoke, and use just vinegar and baking soda for household cleaning and laundry. After thoroughly researching safety measures and finding a skilled dentist, have amalgam fillings safely and gradually removed (see *Personal Care*). For the first year of your program, do not decorate your house or buy new furniture, new flooring, or anything else that could bring toxic chemicals into your home.

Personal Care

Your skin is one of your body's major detoxification organs. It also absorbs everything it comes in contact with, so be very cautious about which products you put on your skin. Unless absolutely necessary, try not to use any soaps, bath foams, shampoos, and so on.

A good rule of thumb is: If you wouldn't eat generous amounts of it, don't put it on your skin! This lesson really hit home for me once after I made a batch of curried fermented vegetables. With my bare hands, I had kneaded the mixture for five to ten minutes. After packing a few small jars, I washed my hands thoroughly. The next day, there was a strong odour emanating from my underarms. It was curry! I had not eaten any for weeks—the curry had passed through my palms and travelled through my entire body. In a similar vein, many people find that coconut oil applied topically increases die-off symptoms. In short, don't underestimate the impact of what you put onto your skin!

You can search online for natural personal care options, including shampoo, deodorant, wound care, cold and flu recovery, cleaning supplies, make up, etc., simply adding the words "natural" or "home remedy" to your need. For example, into your Internet search engine type a phrase such as "cold remedy natural" or "moisturizer home remedy." Earth Clinic (www.earthclinic.com) is a wonderful site that presents consumer experiments and results in the realm of home and natural remedies. Here are some examples of natural solutions to try:

Shampoo alternative: People who never start shampooing may never need to. Except for one or two accidents by well-meaning caregivers, my son's very full head of hair has never been shampooed. It is always clean and bright with a lovely scent. Similarly, many adults who previously used shampoo for years have successfully transitioned to a head full of luxurious locks using no cleansers at all. Those of us intent on applying something to the scalp can try the following approach, which works beautifully for me: Depending on the volume of your hair, separate 1–2 egg yolks from the whites, then rub only the yolks onto your wet hair and scalp. Rinse well. For some, 15 mL (1 tablespoon) of baking soda mixed into 1 cup of water works well and this can be stored in a bottle by your tub. After rinsing with water, you might choose to follow up either of these "shampoos" with a rinse of 15 mL (1 tablespoon) apple cider vinegar per cup of water (it must be diluted to avoid stinging the eyes, but some recipes call for as much as 1 cup of apple cider vinegar to ½ cup of water). An extended application of apple cider vinegar or coconut oil can relieve dandruff and add shine.

Dry skin: Apply the tips presented under *Health Issues: Eczema.*

Sun protection: Avoid sun lotions. Instead, Dr. Campbell-McBride recommends we avoid burns by building sunbathing time gradually, starting with 15 minutes per side, per day, and working up to two hours. Avoid sunbathing on very hot days or during the hottest times of the day (10 AM to 2 PM). The darker your natural pigment, the longer an exposure your skin will prefer. If you get too much sun on your skin, apply homemade yogurt or fermented cream. Many have reported that ingesting cod liver oil regularly, both before and during sun season, helps to prevent sunburns.

Oral hygiene: I highly recommend the use of a Philips Sonicare toothbrush. For me, this gadget has paid for itself several times over in the reduction of dental care required. Also, a GAPS-friendly guide to tooth care can be found at the Natural Dentistry website of Ray Behm, DDS (www.saveyourteeth.com). Navigate to the page titled "The Secret." For those with more involved dental issues, a need for dental intervention, or the presence of amalgam fillings, GAPSters have strongly recommended the following books: *Cure Tooth Decay: Remineralize Cavities and Repair Your Teeth Naturally with Good Food* by Ramiel Nagel (www.curetoothdecay.com), *Radical Medicine: Cutting-Edge Natural Therapies that Treat the Root Causes of Disease* by Dr. Louisa Williams (www.radicalmedicine.com), and *It's All In Your Head: The Link Between Mercury Amalgams and Illness* by Dr. Hal A. Huggins (www.hugginsappliedhealing.com).

Safer products: Products with reduced amounts of chemicals are increasingly available for personal care, cleaning, home renovations, and more. As more consumers commit to purchasing them, prices for these are becoming progressively more affordable. Look for everything from laundry discs to glass water bottles to house paints free of volatile organic compounds (VOCs). These kinds of products can be located in health food stores and online. Specialty, department, and grocery stores also offer options in increasing variety.

Juicing

Much of the information in this section is adapted from the book, *Gut and Psychology Syndrome* (9th edition).

Fresh, home-pressed, raw juices provide necessary vitamins, minerals, amino acids, and live enzymes in an easy to ingest and digest form. The taste also helps people consume more liquid than they otherwise might. All fruit and vegetable juices must be freshly pressed at home, from healthy, ripe, organic produce. Here are some tips:

• You will be starting with a small amount of juice (approximately 45 mL or 3 tablespoons per day) and working up slowly. Thus, you may delay the purchase of a juicer until you have worked up to a significant amount, know that you can tolerate it, and have had a chance to save up for an additional appliance. In the beginning, you can simply blend a small amount of veggies, put the resulting mash into a nutmilk bag or section of cheesecloth, and press the juice through by hand.

- Take juice on an empty stomach, 20–25 minutes before or 2–2½ hours after food.
- The juice can be consumed on its own or mixed with water, whey, or yogurt.
- Incorporating the daily juice into a "GAPS milkshake" as presented in this Guide under *Health Issues: Fat Malabsorption*, will allow the juice to be digested without spikes in blood sugar.
- After working up slowly, aim to include in your Full GAPS program 500 mL (2 cups) of juice (calculated without additional shake ingredients) per day.
- If you do not have diarrhea, continue eating whole vegetables and fruits, too.

Many adults and children enjoy juices made entirely of carrots, carrots and beets, or leafy greens. To satisfy a more fussy palate, create a juice with not more than 50% of its ingredients from the first column in the following chart, and the rest from the second column.

Highly Therapeutic (less than 50% of juice)		Taste Enhancers (over 50% of juice)
Carrot	Dill	Pineapple
Cabbage	Basil	Apple
Celery	Nettle leaves	Orange
Lettuce	Beet tops	Grapefruit
Spinach	Carrot tops	Grapes
Parsley	Cabbage (white or red)	Mango
Beetroot (no more than 5% of total juice)		

Therapeutic Uses

Once you are somewhat familiar with the process of juicing, you may research or invent additional combinations for specific health goals or for general enjoyment (look in juicing books or online for ideas). According to Dr. Campbell-McBride, a combination of carrot, pineapple, and a small amount of beetroot will stimulate stomach acid production, stimulate pancreatic enzyme production, and prepare the digestive system for the coming meal; a mixture of cabbage, apple, and celery will also stimulate digestive enzyme production and cleanse the kidney; leafy vegetables (spinach, lettuce, parsley, dill, carrot, and beet tops) with tomato and lemon added will facilitate heavy metal chelation and infuse the body with magnesium and iron; a combination of carrot, apple, celery, and beetroot will help cleanse the liver; and 5 mL (1 teaspoon) per person of black elderberries added to any juicing combination will enhance immunity.

CHAPTER 4

SUPPLEMENTATION

"Where will I get my B vitamins from?" • *"Without milk from the beginning, where will my child get his calcium from?"*

Many people coming to GAPS are concerned about eating a "restricted" diet. However, even during the most limited phase of the diet (which is too brief to result in deficiencies anyway), GAPS lacks no required nutrient. The B vitamins are found in GAPS' meat (including poultry and fish), asparagus, broccoli, spinach, bananas, dried apricots, dates, figs, milk, eggs, cheese, yogurt, and nuts. Calcium-rich foods include bone broth, sardines, almonds, navy beans, sesame seeds, broccoli, and dark green leafy vegetables (e.g., turnip greens, dandelion greens, kale, spinach, and seaweed). Organ meats are an excellent source of iron.

Indeed, nutrient-dense, properly prepared food in its whole form should be our primary source of nutrients. This noted, Dr. Campbell-McBride does recommend a handful of bottled foods: probiotics, up to three oils, stomach acid for some people, and case-specific supplementation for some people.

Supplement timing: Start Intro with no supplements, then introduce each supplement one at a time, at any point during or after Intro. Within this Guide's *Stages of Intro* section, I offer tips about when during Intro one might start these.

Supplement forms and ingredients: Choose supplements free of ingredients that might aggravate the gut. For oils, liquids (versus gelcaps) may reduce the amount of additional ingredients and are preferable, but whatever form you can ingest is fine. Supplements can also be compounded, free of additional ingredients, at your local pharmacy. Regardless of the supplement's form or lack of extraneous ingredients, not all supplements are tolerated by all people. Some may react, for example, to cod liver oil. When a GAPS supplement is not tolerated, even by the "low and slow" method presented under *Probiotic FAQs: How much should I start with and increase by?*, leave it out of your program. Consider retesting the supplement after every few months of additional healing.

Supplement shopping: Dr. Campbell-McBride does not make any specific brand recommendations. Much of the detailed supplement information below, including product suggestions, has been provided by International Nutrition. This company-specific information is included because, for many of us, researching brands that would prove GAPS-friendly is simply more than we can cope with doing while coming to grips with the rest of the information. International Nutrition offers GAPS books, supplements, and more via the GAPS Diet website (www.GAPSdiet.com) for Canada and U.S. orders, and via NuTriVene (www.nutrivene.com) for orders from all other countries. If you contact them directly with your request, International Nutrition can provide samples (e.g., a few capsules) of the non-liquid supplements it sells. This will allow you to determine whether you have a sensitivity to that particular product before investing in it. But it is equally fine to go to your local health food store, naturopathic clinic, or elsewhere and choose other brands which meet the criteria—as detailed subsequently—for each recommended supplement. Some businesses will provide refunds on supplements that a customer reacts to or does not noticeably benefit from (before shopping, ask for the store's refund policy on supplements).

Supplement questions: For any questions about supplement ingredients, dosing, or contraindications, contact the supplement's manufacturer, sales outlet, and/or your health care provider.

Recommended Supplements

The following supplementation protocol is to be taken in conjunction with—not in place of—the diet. The recommended supplements for GAPS patients are:

- Essential fatty acids in the form of a nut/seed oil;
- Essential fatty acids in the form of fish oil;[1]
- Vitamin A in the form of cod liver oil;[1]
- Betaine HCL with pepsin (in some cases);
- Vitamin and mineral supplements(in some cases); and
- An effective, therapeutic-strength probiotic.

Essential Fatty Acids

Dr. Campbell-McBride recommends that GAPS patients receive more eicosapentaenoic acid (EPA) than docosahexaenoic acid (DHA) through two types of oils: fish and nut/seed. These are to be kept in opaque bottles and refrigerated. There are no toxic levels for these oils.

A nut/seed oil should have more omega-3 than omega-6 fatty acids (the exact ratios are not critical). One option provided by International Nutrition is Barlean's Lignan Omega Twin. Start with a few drops added to cold or warm food. For a child younger than 18 months of age, slowly build the dose to 5–10 mL (1–2 teaspoons) per day. For a child older than 18 months, build the dose to 15–45 mL (1–3 tablespoons) per day. Adults can start with 5 mL (1 teaspoon) per day and slowly work up to 60–75 mL (4–5 tablespoons) per day.

---

[1] Note: Dr. Campbell-McBride recommends that fish oil and cod liver oil not be introduced to a person with symptoms of involuntary movements, such as tics or seizures.

For the fish oil, one option provided by International Nutrition is Nordic Naturals® ProEFA®. Start with a few drops added to cold or warm (not hot) food. For a child younger than 24 months, slowly build the dose to 5 mL (1 teaspoon) per day. For a child older than 24 months, slowly build the dose to 5–15 mL (1–3 teaspoons) per day. For an adult, slowly build the dose to 15–20 mL (3–4 teaspoons) per day. Again, fish oil is not recommended for people with symptoms of involuntary movements, such as tics or seizures.

Cod Liver Oil

Again, cod liver oil is not recommended for a person with symptoms of involuntary movements, such as tics or seizures.

Vitamin A is critical to digestion, but people with digestive problems cannot make full use of the vitamin A found in most supplements. A natural form of vitamin A found in cod liver oil seems to be the best form for people following the GAPS program. One option is BLUE ICE Fermented Cod Liver Oil (CLO) by Green Pasture. Fermented CLO is far easier to digest than regular CLO, thus absorption is increased and the nutrients are easier to assimilate. It contains 2½ times more of the therapeutic vitamins A and D, and uses no heat during production; therefore, the precious enzymes, vitamins, and other nutrients that would usually be destroyed by food processing are retained. Fermentation not only concentrates nutrition, but it also makes that nutrition more bioavailable. BLUE ICE Fermented CLO is a tremendous source of EPA, DHA, Vitamins A, D, E, and K, Omega 3, 6, 7, and 9, as well as Price Factor X (vitamin K). The manufacturer of BLUE ICE Fermented CLO recommends taking it with high-vitamin butter oil (e.g., the X-FACTOR high-vitamin butter oils) for maximum effectiveness. If you choose to use butter oil, introduce it when or after you introduce ghee to your diet. Dr. Campbell-McBride suggests taking the fermented CLO in the amounts recommended by its manufacturer, with children taking half the adult dose. Dr. Campbell-McBride recommends that pregnant or lactating women take double the usual adult dose. As always, find out from your GAPS-friendly health practitioner what levels of supplementation are ideal for your age and circumstance. Again, any supplement can trigger a reaction, so start with a small amount and work up slowly. If the supplement is tolerated, Dr. Campbell-McBride also notes that the therapeutic dose can be doubled for the first few weeks upon reaching it. If fermented CLO is not available to you and you must use a non-fermented product, Dr. Campbell-McBride recommends using one with a ratio of approximately ten units of vitamin A to one unit of vitamin D, dosed at the amounts recommended by the product's manufacturer for a child, pregnant or lactating woman, or other adult. CLO can trigger wakefulness in some people, so take it in the morning rather than within a few hours of bedtime.

Stomach Acid (Betaine HCL with Pepsin)

People with abnormal gut flora almost without exception also have low stomach acid production. Toxins produced by overgrowth of *Candida, Clostridia,* and other pathogens severely reduce secretion of stomach acid. Often, this issue can be resolved by the simple steps offered in this Guide under *Health Issues: Heartburn, Reflux, and Indigestion.* Dr. Campbell-McBride recommends introducing betaine HCL if an adult is burping excessively after food, or if a child is burping excessively after food after some time on the program. Initially, it is to be taken after the meal (to avoid burning the stomach). After a good amount of healing has taken place, the person can start taking it at the beginning of the meal. The most physiological preparation available is betaine HCl with pepsin. Since many of the betaine HCL with pepsin preparations on the market may not be suitable for children because of the strength, International Nutrition asked Dr. Campbell-McBride what the ideal proportions would be for children. Dr. Campbell-McBride suggested a capsule size of 150–200 mg of betaine HCL and 900 National Formulary (NF) units (approximately 3–4 mg) of pepsin. International Nutrition offers the betaine HCL with pepsin according to these specifications.

If Intro and the tips presented under *Health Issues: Heartburn, Reflux, and Indigestion* do not sufficiently resolve poor digestion in a child, and the use of betaine HCL is being considered, see Dr. Campbell-McBride's book *Gut and Psychology Syndrome,* as well as her FAQ document, or consult with the company providing your supplement, for dosing amounts for children and adults per each individual's circumstances.

Other Supplements

It is advised to begin the program with just food and then add the GAPS-specific supplements. Add in additional therapies and supplements only when the body has had several months to heal or if there is an indication of urgent need, such as in those cases described by Dr. Campbell-McBride in her FAQ document, in which she suggests a specific bedtime dose of 5-Hydroxytryptophan (5-HTP) when a child's sleep or need for increased calm indicates, pancreatic (digestive) enzymes in the case of chronic fatigue syndrome or fibromyalgia, ox bile in the case of fat malabsorption issues, and so on. Search within that document for the diagnosis or symptom of concern to you.

Your local osteopath, nutritionist, or naturopath—preferably one familiar with GAPS—may also be an excellent resource in the matter of additional supplementation. For a person with Down's syndrome, a wonderful resource is International Nutrition, mentioned previously. For a person with impairment of thought, perception, mood, or clarity (e.g., bipolar disorder, OCD, AD(H)D, depression, or anxiety), a good resource is Truehope (www.truehope.com). People with any of these disorders or symptoms of challenged aging, alcoholism, psychosis, schizophrenia, or Parkinson's, the Orthomolecular Vitamin Information Centre (www.orthomolecularvitamincentre.com) may be of assistance. The latter is dedicated to the work of the late Dr. Abram Hoffer, mentioned in my personal story, who advised his clients to enjoy a GAPS-like, nutrient-dense diet free of allergens and complemented with specific doses of vitamins. All of these resources offer services to people throughout the world.

Probiotics

The topic of probiotics brings up many questions, and a random approach to incorporating them creates many issues. Please be sure to review this entire section before introducing them. Following the tips offered in the following Q&A can save you from unnecessary frustration, discomfort, and expense.

Probiotic FAQs

"What are some sources of probiotics?" Probiotics are found in fermented foods such as homemade whey, kefir, yogurt, and fermented vegetables as well as in commercial supplies (i.e., capsules or powder).

"What if I can't afford a therapeutic dose of a commercial probiotic?" Many people experience excellent healing by using copious home-ferments daily. However, if you are not yet committed to creating and ingesting regular doses of fermented vegetables, fermented fish, yogurt, kefir, fermented coconut water, etc., the expense of a commercial probiotic will be necessary and worthwhile. You can also mix-and-match the homemade and commercial options, taking a smaller or less frequent amount of homemade options while also taking a moderate dose of a commercial probiotic. Regardless of the source of probiotic you choose, be sure to start with just one source at a time, and build the dose of each one slowly.

"Will I heal without a therapeutic dose of a commercial probiotic?" Whether or not you are taking a commercial probiotic, it is impossible for anyone to make projections about your GAPS results. However, at least one mother on one of our online support lists has seen tremendous healing in her son even though he cannot take any supplement, including any bottled probiotic.

"Will a probiotic help me even if I'm not doing the diet?" In her book *Gut and Psychology Syndrome* (9th edition), Dr. Campbell-McBride said: "Adhering to the diet is absolutely essential [while taking the probiotics]. If you carry on feeding [the] pathogens in the gut with sugar and processed carbohydrates then the probiotic will not have much chance of helping you."

"I'm intolerant to casein/lactose. Some commercial probiotics contain traces of milk. Should I take it or not?" Most of us are unable to process casein until we have been on GAPS for some time, and most of us are unable to process lactose even after being on GAPS for many months. Despite this, most of us are fine with commercial probiotics that contain either of these. In most cases, those who have reacted to a commercial probiotic started with relatively large amounts (despite the repeated recommendations to start with a tiny amount and work up). Follow the instructions for a "low and slow" introduction and increase, as presented subsequently within this section. Also, feel free to try various brands: International Nutrition can provide a sample of at least one probiotic, and many businesses will provide a refund on supplements if you react to them or notice no benefit. Finally, a simple alternative is offered under the question: *"How do I know if I'm reacting to a filler or having die-off?"*

"Some commercial probiotics include Bifidus, which Elaine Gottschall said to avoid. Should I not use these products?" Conflicting reports that Elaine Gottschall had accessed gave her concern regarding a potential for Bifidus to overgrow, thus she declared Bifidus "SCD illegal." Dr. Campbell-McBride feels it is beneficial to use a wide range of strains, including Bifidus, and most people coming to GAPS report no issues with these. While some people feel that Bifidus and other strains of bacteria have been specifically helpful in their healing, some SCDers have said that Bifidus is problematic for them, causing chronic loose stools. If you feel that Bifidus or any other strain is a problem or could be a problem for you, feel free to start with a probiotic which includes only strains you are currently comfortable with. After some months of healing, evaluate whether more strains could be included in your personal program. In the meantime, a simple alternative is offered under the question: *"How do I know if I'm reacting to a filler or having die-off?"*

"So many of the commercial probiotics include maltodextrin. I thought we weren't supposed to have maltodextrin." You're right; GAPS people should generally not have maltodextrin. However, Dr. Campbell-McBride feels that, for most people, the amount of maltodextrin in a quality probiotic is not enough to worry about. However, some people may find they react to it. A simple alternative is offered under the question: *"How do I know if I'm reacting to a filler or having die-off?"*

"How do I know if I'm reacting to a filler or having die-off?" Just as with food reactions versus die-off, the answer is, "Generally, you don't know." If you have any concerns, you can start with an "SCD legal" probiotic, such as scdophilus from GI Pro Health (www.giprohealth.com).

"What effects will I notice?" The intensity of effects will depend very much on the dose you start at or increase by. Be sure to read the information, presented subsequently, under "How much bottled probiotic should I take?" and "How much should I start with and increase by?" Once you have determined an appropriate amount to start with or increase by, watch for any "die-off" symptoms upon every new dose, including but not limited to fatigue, nausea, bloating, diarrhea, constipation, low-grade fever, headache, flu-like symptoms, or behavioural changes. If any of these are experienced, they should be neither terribly uncomfortable nor persistent. Mild die-off will often resolve within a day or two without intervention. If symptoms are bothersome, reduce your dose to your last tolerated level (or just barely more than that) and, in the meantime, implement one or more of the die-off relief strategies offered in this Guide, such as die-off relief baths, naps, or activated charcoal. Whether die-off is mild or intense, once it has resolved, you might like to "cruise" at your newest dose for a while, enjoying the break from die-off. Increase the dose when you are ready to experience die-off again.

If upon starting or increasing a probiotic, you experience no noticeable die-off, still allow a full week at that daily dose before increasing the dose further (the effects may prove cumulative over the week), then increase the dose by a very small amount.

Some people feel no noticeable effect from any dose of probiotics. If this is the case for you, you may feel frustrated and wonder if you are throwing your money away. In this situation, I propose that you may still be benefiting from a therapeutic dose—your body may simply not provide an obvious response. (For some people, this happens with the diet aspect, too. In these cases, when the diet or probiotics are stopped, the person's health noticeably decreases. This is the only indication these folks have that the diet or a given supplement was indeed making a significant difference.) You might also want to try other brands, to see if another brings an obvious response.

"How much bottled probiotic should I take?" Every commercial probiotic offers a different amount of live bacteria per capsule, so it is not possible to present a starting dose in "number of capsules" because that will depend on which probiotic you choose to use. Although the therapeutic dose is different for everyone, Dr. Campbell-McBride presents the following as a starting point for consideration. Alongside these numbers are offered capsule amounts using the example of Bio-Kult, which has a live unit count of two billion probiotic microorganisms per capsule. You can calculate the equivalent for any brand of your choice.

Age	Recommended Dosage
0–12 months	1–2 billion bacterial cells per day (½–1 capsule of Bio-Kult)
1–2 years	2–4 billion bacterial cells per day (1–2 capsules of Bio-Kult)
2–4 years	4–8 billion bacterial cells per day (2–4 capsules of Bio-Kult)
4–10 years	8–12 billion bacterial cells per day (4–6 capsules of Bio-Kult)
12–16 years	12–15 billion bacterial cells per day (6–8 capsules of Bio-Kult)
17 years and older	15–20 billion bacterial cells per day (8–10 capsules of Bio-Kult)

Again, every bottled probiotic has its own potency, so you need to read the bacterial count on a given bottle before determining how many capsules or grams of that particular product will achieve the desired goal.

Dr. Campbell-McBride notes that once you have reached the therapeutic dose, it should be maintained for approximately six months. She states that it takes at least this long to remove the pathogenic flora and to start re-establishing normal gut flora. Again, for minimal die-off and maximum progress, one must start with a fraction of the therapeutic dose (see the following section). Generally, a person will start with a tiny amount of a homemade or commercial probiotic and then work up very slowly. When you notice healing and are satisfied that you are continuing to progress in health, maintain that level of probiotic. There is no benefit in going over the amounts listed, which would simply bring unnecessary expense (and possibly physical overwhelm). Over time, continue increasing your homemade ferments. After six months on the therapeutic dose, with homemade ferments gradually increased in the meantime, start to slowly decrease the commercial probiotic to a maintenance dose; this is usually half of a therapeutic one but with sufficient homemade ferments included, even less may be needed. To determine your maintenance dose, do this: slowly decrease the amount of commercial probiotic you are taking (e.g., by ¼ capsule per week) and watch for any changes in your health. For example, reducing these too quickly triggered both my son and me to stop having bowel movements. Eventually, your maintenance dose may be achievable through fermented foods alone.

"How much should I start with and increase by?" Whatever amount you think is low, start with—and increase by—far less! Some people will need 6 months or more to reach a therapeutic dose.

For an adult whose symptoms are not severe and who is not generally sensitive to supplements and medications, I recommend starting with 500 million live cells or less per day, divided into a morning and evening dose. Again, every commercial probiotic offers a different number of live cells. If using Bio-Kult®, this suggested starting dose is achieved with 1/4 capsule per day (1/8th of a capsule in the morning and 1/8th of a capsule in the evening). Primal Defense Ultra®, on the other hand, offers 5 billion live cells per capsule, so the starting dose would be achieved with 1/10th of a capsule of Primal Defense Ultra® (1/20th capsule in the morning and 1/20th capsule in the evening).

It is important to consider carefully the live cell count offered by the probiotic you are choosing to use, and to determine what portion of the capsule offers 500 million live cells or less. (Google's search engine will do the math for you. Type in the amount of live cells offered in one capsule divided by 500 million, e.g., "2 billion divided by 500 million". Divide the capsule by the resulting number.) Take half of that amount in the morning and half in the evening. You will not be able to measure out precisely this portion; an estimate will be fine. When using a portion of a capsule, open it up, tip out the portion needed, re-close the capsule, put the capsule in a tightly closed jar, and put the jar in the fridge. Continue accessing portions from this capsule until it is empty, then start with a new one.

If die-off is tolerable (or not even noticeable), maintain your initial dose for at least 1 week before considering an increase. Once at least 1 week has passed, and any die-off has completely resolved, you might increase your dose by that amount again (e.g., by ¼ capsule of Bio-Kult® to a total of ½ capsule per day).

For a child or a very ill or very sensitive adult, I recommend starting with even less and increasing at a slower pace. Continuing to use Bio-Kult® in this example, one might start with one-tenth of a capsule or less per day, increasing by just one-tenth of a capsule after a week or more. (This portion of a Bio-Kult® capsule offers approximately 200 million live cells. Again, start with the proportion of your chosen capsule that supplies that amount or less.) Some experience intense die-off with even the smallest amount of probiotic—including an SCD-legal one. They may have to take just the amount that the tip of a vertically inserted knife picks up, or dilute the powder and take only a drop of that liquid. The "low and slow" method of introduction for supplements may be key for these folks:

- Day 1: Starting dose of your choice, just once in the day. Ensure a lower amount (e.g., 50 million live cells or less) by using a lower-dose probiotic, taken in any of the following ways: one pinch of powder, or the amount that fits on the tip of a vertically-inserted butter knife, or that amount diluted in water with one sip taken.
- Day 2: None
- Day 3: If no die-off is experienced, double the Day 1 dose by taking the same dose again, but in both the morning and in the evening.
- Day 4: None
- Day 5: If no die-off is experienced, increase the morning dose only.
- Continue to increase every second day until light die-off is experienced.
- When die-off is experienced, stay at that dose until the die-off resolves.

Regardless of your starting point, as you progress you may find you can incorporate a larger increase—perhaps of ¼ capsule, then ½ capsule, then 1 capsule—every four days or so until you have reached the therapeutic dose. However, do not rush this process. Intense die-off can be triggered by relatively small increases, or be noticed only after a week or so of a new dose. It is far more comfortable—and more effective—to move slowly and surely than it is to jump forward, suffer intense die-off, work backward, then start the process over. Increasing once a week is easy to remember and plenty fast enough.

"The info sheet from the company through which I ordered my Bio-Kult said to give my ten-year-old six capsules in week 6." Unless specifically indicated as applicable to GAPS, information sheets distributed with probiotics relate to general use and do not necessarily apply to people doing GAPS.

"I give my baby eight billion bacterial cells per day. Do you think this is fine?" This is far more than is needed by a baby doing GAPS. This can also cause uncomfortable gas, bloating, and die-off. It also involves an unnecessary degree of expense. Please see the previous questions and answers in this section.

"I recently increased my probiotic from four capsules to five. I feel funny." In a probiotic with a high count of live cells per capsule, an increase of one capsule can be far too much. When I increased mine early on from 1 capsule to 2, I had intense die-off: it's simply too much, too quickly. Drop the dose back to the amount you were most recently tolerating well, and work up very slowly.

"I'm on Week 2 of Intro and having every day: 1 cup of kefir, 2 capsules of probiotics, and 3 teaspoons of juice from fermented vegetables with each meal. Why am I not feeling well?" This is an enormous amount of probiotic content for this early point in your healing program. Stop or drastically reduce all probiotics and start them again gently and slowly, one source at a time, as detailed in this Guide.

"When should I take my probiotic?" In most cases, take your probiotic with or shortly after food. An exception to this is if you are including betaine HCL in your program. If including betaine HCL in your program, take the betaine with meals and take your probiotic at a different time, such as first thing in the morning and just before bed. With either approach, take half your daily dose of the probiotic at some point in the morning and half at some point in the evening.

"In terms of bottled probiotics, what do I look for when shopping?" No one commercial probiotic is recommended more than another. In her book *Gut and Psychology Syndrome,* Dr. Campbell-McBride sets out her recommendations for probiotics in general. Essentially, she likes to see:

- As many different species of beneficial bacteria as possible;
- A mixture of strains from different groups (e.g., lactobacilli; bifidobacteria; and soil-based organisms);
- At least eight billion live bacterial cells per gram;
- Each batch tested for strength and bacterial composition, with the manufacturer willing to publish the results;
- No enteric coating; and
- No fillers that would bother a person.

Most commercial probiotics have SCD-illegal ingredients, such as maltodextrin, fructooligosaccharides (FOS), or oat grass. Any time you choose a product with an SCD-illegal component, you risk a reaction to that ingredient. This is something you have to weigh, research, and/or test for yourself. Also, when researching options, note that some bottled probiotics have a much higher potency than others, so you need to read the bacterial count on a given bottle before determining its true cost, as well as the amount needed. For example, to achieve therapeutic doses, one would need many, many capsules per day of Garden of Life's Primal Defense® Probiotic Formula, but only a few of Primal Defense® ULTRA Ultimate Probiotic Formula. That's how varied bacterial counts can be from bottle to bottle, even when produced by the same company.

"What if I'm positive I have an overgrowth of one bacteria and/or an undersupply of another?" Upon consideration of all of the above recommendations, feel free to supplement with the bacteria of your choice.

CHAPTER 5

MONTHS 1–3: PREPARING FOR FULL GAPS/INTRO

This phase was initially developed in response to the many folks who, like me, burst into tears after attempting to start the SCD and/or GAPS "today." For those with a sensitive system that may react to even the single step of removing grains, or those who have a lot on their plate already, or those who have not yet cooked whole foods from scratch, or those whose lifestyle is quite far removed from the one proposed, the following will be of great assistance. However, even for those coming to GAPS from an already excellent diet or from a simple lifestyle rich in homemade foods, this phase can still make your GAPS journey immensely easier—you might simply proceed through it in one month versus three months.

This section will:

- Walk you gently through a transition to avoid physical, emotional, or psychological overwhelm;
- Help you source key tools and ingredients so that you are ready for Full GAPS and Intro;
- Give you a chance to practice new recipes, especially the foundational ones required for Intro and Full GAPS;
- Allow your body to adjust slowly to powerful foods; and
- Minimize major withdrawal symptoms.

You may experience significant changes in your body even with this gentle transition! Changes may occur upon adding powerful foods, such as broth or kefir, or upon reducing common sugars. Although a gentle transition (especially one that focuses on progressively adding in nutrient-dense foods rather than suddenly removing all the poorer ones) will help to minimize any discomfort that may be felt in the process of dietary changes, you may still experience some degree of these. If during this transition you do experience changes in your body, review the information under *Months 4–6: What to Expect in Intro*. Your experience may be discussed there.

Many people come to GAPS from WAPF or the "caveman diet" or another excellent, nutrient-dense diet. For several months or years they have been eating a diet that has many overlaps with GAPS, or one that at the very least includes a hefty population of natural ferments. Thus, I am often asked: "Since I've eaten an excellent diet—full of fats, bone broth, and kefir—for so many months already, can I skip Intro and/or continue my homemade probiotic foods at their current levels and/or simply remove the few things that are not recommended for GAPS patients?" My answer is that although your excellent diet will definitely position you for an easier psychological and physical transition to GAPS, your body will notice the difference. Doing Intro will still bring great gains, and the cleansing/healing effects will likely bring up reactions even to your previously incorporated levels of probiotic foods. Please do GAPS as outlined. Your experience with eating a cleaner, more nutrient-dense diet will provide you with an easier transition and possibly faster healing, but for best results follow all the steps and tips.

The only people who might consider jumping from their current diet directly to Intro are those who will otherwise require immediate institutionalization (such as Kevin, whose story is presented in the *More Stories* section of this Guide) or those with severe intestinal issues, such as Crohn's disease or ulcerative colitis. For these, the relief and benefits experienced in early Intro may strongly outweigh the discomfort otherwise triggered by jumping right in. Even if you fall into one of these categories, please still read this whole section through carefully—it includes tips helpful for your overall journey. If you do have a serious bowel disorder, the *Health Issues: Severe Intestinal Issues* section of this Guide will be of additional help to you.

Program Tools

The essentials for GAPS are few. While certain appliances can make some aspects of the program much easier, they are not critical to own. Some people love to use a crock pot for slow simmering while at work, for example. If you have one, feel free to use it. If you don't have one, a crock pot is not necessary—feel free to save the money for food. Similarly, a handheld or immersion blender is lovely for blending soups right in the pot or making a quick applesauce, but it's not a necessary tool. For your budget's sake, opt for just the items that are crucial for you. The first list presented below is that of items I recommend having on hand from the start. The second list can be explored according to need, interest, and financial ability. For updates to these lists, further details on any given item, active product links, and other people's comments, please see GAPSguide.com.

Please note that within this book, amounts of supplies and recipes are based on one adult plus one child. Adjust all amounts to match your own family's needs.

Essential Items

- **Activated Charcoal (capsule or liquid):** This remedy, available at most health and drug stores, brought me great relief during a too-intense die-off (I only had to use it once). Use as directed on the bottle or by your health practitioner.

- **Baking Soda:** I love it for deodorizing, cleaning, detox baths, and much more.

- **Casserole Dish:** For casseroles, savoury pies, and so on. A lid may come in handy, but is not needed for most recipes.

- **Colander and/or Sieve:** I use a colander for draining tiny bones, etc., out of a broth and for draining and rinsing soaked nuts. I use a sieve for draining and rinsing small seeds, such as sesame seeds.

- **Cutting Board.**

- **Enema Kit:** Please see this Guide's section *Detoxification: Enemas.*

- **Epsom Salts:** These make a wonderfully soothing detox (and/or constipation-relieving) bath.

- **Food:** In a sense, this goes without saying. I've explicitly included it here to emphasize that this needs to be a priority. Before delving too far into manufactured goods and supplements, be sure to establish sound eating habits. Food is incredibly healing. It is irreplaceable. Let it demonstrate its abilities before you explore add-ons.

- **Food Storage Containers:** It is helpful to have a variety, ranging in size from 250 mL (1 cup) to 1 litre (4 cups). These will hold leftovers, vegetables cut and frozen at home, broth portioned for a day or week, and so on. I use a mix of plastic (for school snacks) and glass (for foods transitioning from the stove to the fridge or freezer).

- **Insulated Food Containers:** Correctly conditioned before each use, these can be used to keep cold foods cold or hot foods hot. I use one from the Thermos® brand "Steel Commuter" line. I chose one that held 470 mL (approximately 2 cups), because this was the largest one available that was still simple in design. I chose a wide-mouth, perfect cylinder so that I could scoop all the way to the bottom and also fit my entire hand in to clean it. I chose one with no parts besides body and lid (i.e., no handle, straw, or built-in spoon) so that it would be easy to clean and so that it would have fewer parts that could break. I have four of these. For a picnic, we fill two with drinking water and two with our meal. Some people avoid stainless steel (due to concerns about potential leaching of nickel or cadmium), so they might opt for a glass-lined version—but be aware that some companies offering "glass" containers may line the glass with non-removable plastic.

- **Jars with Lids:** I like wide-mouth glass mason jars, so that I can see what I've stored in them, fill them easily, retrieve food from them with a cooking spoon, and fit my hand in to clean them well. For ghee, leftovers, larger storage, and fermenting, I like to have at least eight 1–2 litre (1–2 quart) jars. I buy canning jars from thrift shops and buy new lids from any department store. When freezing food in glass jars, fill them only three-quarters full to prevent breakage.

- **Journal:** Whether in the form of a calendar, loose-leaf paper in a binder, or a computer spreadsheet, many people find it helpful to keep a simple, daily record of date, item added, bath taken, supplements ingested, and signs of struggle or improvement.

- **Knife:** When I started cooking up a storm, a friend gave me an awesome knife that she found at a thrift shop: a J.A. Henckels International (www.j-a-henckels.com) 200 mm (8 inch) No Stain Model 31161. Large and heavy, it practically does the work for me, even on a raw butternut squash! A good knife can make all the difference to your ease, energy, and happiness in the kitchen. I cannot emphasize this enough. Don't skimp here. Others strongly recommend a 250 mm (10 inch) chef's knife, insisting that if we like the 200 mm (8 inch), we will be ecstatic over the self-employment leanings of a 250 mm (10 inch)!

- **Knife Sharpener:** As clumsy and inattentive as I can be at times, I didn't feel safe with any until I met the J.A. Henckels Twinsharp Knife Sharpener. It is safe, simple, fast, and super effective. I press my knife through it every second or third cooking session and I have a brand new knife!

- **Labels:** Because you will be observing the effects that various ingredients have on your body, it will be important to have all frozen and refrigerated foods thoroughly labelled. A label may be made of masking tape, removable white stickers from a stationery store, and so on.

- **Large Pot with Lid:** This versatile item is critical for the big batches of broth and soup you will be making during Intro (or every day throughout the entire healing program for a big family), but it works equally well for a single serving of sole and onions, for example. Mine holds approximately 8 litres (32 cups or 8 quarts). Although some folks avoid stainless steel over concerns of nickel or cadmium potentially leaching, I use stainless steel happily. Cast iron, or glass that is stovetop safe, are also good options. Two favourites within the GAPS community are the Le Creuset stock pot and the Rival Crockpot Versaware Pro. Mine is a simple, low-cost, department store brand.

- **Nut Milk Bag or Cheesecloth:** Available from most health food stores, a nut milk bag is helpful for dripping yogurt, covering a jar of kefir, straining the juice from blended vegetables or nuts, and so on. A section of cheesecloth can also serve most of these purposes, but a nut milk bag can also be hung from a cupboard door, which is how I do most of my dripping.

- **Recipes:** There are hundreds of GAPS-friendly recipes available online for free. Folks that prefer recipes collated, indexed, and printed will enjoy any one or more of the recipe books available in electronic or hardcopy format. See this Guide's section *Recipes: More Essentials–More Recipes for Intro and Beyond.*

- **Thermometers (for meat and yogurt):** These allow you to ensure safety (meats) and maximum effectiveness (yogurts). Be sure to get ones that can be recalibrated and then do this regularly.

- **Yogurt Maker:** Please refer to this Guide's *Yogurt* recipe for a wide variety of equipment options, including homemade ones.

Subsequent Items

Any of the following items can be incorporated as your commitment, healing, needs, intuition, and/or budget determine.

- **Blender:** This can be as simple and affordable as a stick (immersion) blender, or as powerful as a food processor. I primarily use a Cuisinart Smart Stick Hand Blender with Whisk and Chopper Attachment, which allows me to whip up a soup, pâté, or dip in seconds, then detach and quickly clean the active part. I use this up to three times per day.

- **Cleaner Water:** The cleanliness of your water supply depends upon where you live and the system used to access it. Some municipalities have state-of-the-art systems that provide very clean water for their residents. While some people can maintain good health relying just on their local supply, others are more sensitive to elements within their water. Your water filtration needs will vary according to the water available to you and your level of sensitivity to anything it might contain. Your water filtration options will also range greatly depending on a number of factors, such as whether you rent a room or own a house. A filter can be as simple as a carbon cap on a faucet or as comprehensive as a whole-house system set up at your household water's point of entry. As your budget allows, start with filtered water for your drinking, then bathing, then showering, then cooking, then for all other uses.

- **Dehydrator:** A popular model is the Excalibur® 9-Tray with Timer (www.excaliburdehydrator.com). In my chronically cool and drafty house, this machine is super helpful for making yogurt (I set it to 40°C or 105°F and achieve 41°C or 106°F) as well as for maintaining the correct temperature for fermenting vegetables. Others enjoy it for making zucchini chips, dehydrating cookies, re-crisping soaked almonds, and so on. I also had success with these activities; however, after some initial experiments, I found myself skipping any activity that wasn't absolutely necessary to my GAPS program. Thus, this machine may or may not be important to you, depending on what you love to do. While I continue to love the simplicity and tidiness of the dehydrator for my ferments, there are lower-cost options—as detailed in this Guide's *Yogurt* recipe—for maintaining fermentation temperatures.

- **Food Processor:** This machine makes easy work of chopping or mincing large amounts of vegetables (including for ferments) and making nut butter, ice cream, and so on.

- **Grinders:** Available in various sizes, grinders can crush peppercorns, pulverize seeds, make nut flours, and so on.

- **Homogenizer:** This tool makes food such as nut butters and ice creams smooth. A food processor, or a quality juicer such as the Champion (www.championjuicer.com) which incorporates a homogenizing function, can often serve this function.

- **Juicer:** Juicing is an important part of the GAPS protocol. Many different juicers are available. Higher quality ones transfer less heat to the produce, allowing it to retain more vitamins, enzymes, and minerals. But spending hundreds of dollars on an especially high-end juicer may be beyond your family's budget, while providing perhaps negligible difference over the health benefits found through a lower-end one. Also, juice is introduced slowly, starting with a very small amount. Thus, you might start by simply blending vegetables in a strong food processor, then pressing the juices out through a nut milk bag or cheesecloth. If the juices prove to be tolerated, consider getting the lowest cost juicer that meets your personal priorities (e.g., quietness, ease of cleaning, portability, and storage). If you find yourself committed enough to use this at least once a week (and preferably daily) for a full year, you might decide to upgrade. Personally, after experimenting with using and cleaning some of the best, I did not ultimately find one I liked enough to own. I continue to search for a small, silent, quick-to-clean juicer.

- **Pan:** Almost anything can be cooked in the pot listed previously, but a pan is handy for cooking smaller dishes, frying eggs, reheating leftovers, and so on. I use a cast iron pan.

- **Steamer Basket:** I use a collapsible one that fits into any pot. I steam squash, greens—you name it.

- **Supplements:** In addition to the diet, and in the ratios prescribed by Dr. Campbell-McBride, I initially found the essential fatty acids (EFAs) critical to remaining depression-free. (After healing, I found I remained depression-free even while forgetting to take these.) Also, a commercial probiotic (Bio-Kult, in our case) successfully triggered die-off. Earlier in the program, I found that when we skipped the probiotic for several days, my son and I both stopped having bowel movements (much of stool is used bacteria). I have not noticed specific results with the fermented cod liver oil, but I was pleased that the taste did indeed become bearable to me over time (my son, on the other hand, has loved it right from his very first taste and frequently asks for more).

- **Tea Tree Oil:** It has so many uses. Among them, a drop in shampoo can relieve dandruff and a drop in the laundry will disinfect clothing.

- **Your Preference:** Your needs are unique, so only you can determine what is key for you beyond the basics. Do you have a very large family, such that chopping vegetables is very time-consuming? If so, a food processor might be worth the cost. Does your family adore spaghetti-style noodles and curly fries? In this case, a $40 spiralizer may prove to be a good investment. Is crushing peppercorns with a wooden spoon (as I did for years) a bother? A pepper grinder could be a good fit. Do you love to make things from scratch, preserve, and create different textures? While definitely not needed by everyone, a dehydrator might be a boon to you.

If space, finances, or overwhelm is an issue, begin your journey with just the essentials, and enhance your kitchen as your needs dictate and your budget allows.

The Steps

If you feel overwhelmed before or at any point during the following process, feel free to do one step, then take a break for a few days or weeks, then move on to the subsequent step.

1. Do not do GAPS. Not today at least, and not this month for that matter. For most people, even those who have done very similar programs, GAPS is a

huge change. It will be felt physically, emotionally, psychologically, and relationally. The impact the change will have on your life must not be underestimated. Your schedule, social life, physical capacity and energy, emotions, relationships, and thoughts will all be affected. A slow and steady transition will support you through the emotional, psychological, and physical changes inherent to the program. Plan to be 100% GAPS no sooner than four weeks from now. Depending on your starting point, 8–12 weeks may be a better fit.

2. Read this entire Guide through before taking a single step. Most of us are so eager to heal that we jump right into Intro or Full GAPS within a week or two of finding out about the program. Ironically, this approach can dramatically slow our healing, not to mention bring us much frustration and unnecessary expense. I have spent literally hundreds of hours developing this Guide, based on the experiences, errors, and successes of many people. My goal is to help you develop a personal approach that is kind to your mind, your body, your relationships, and your wallet. Give yourself this gift: read the Guide through, and then follow the steps as presented.

3. If you know or suspect that you have any serious health condition, such as diabetes, heart problems, and so on, connect with an appropriate health practitioner (e.g., general physician, naturopath, osteopath, or dietitian) about the information presented in this book or about general contraindications for your condition or age. Because everything we eat, drink, bathe in, and apply to our skin can have a dramatic impact on one's physical and mental state, it is important to discuss with your health care practitioner any contraindications between your current health condition and the information presented here. Similarly, seek guidance when applying information to anyone in your care, such as an infant, small child, infirm adult, or an elderly person. For example, if a salt bath is contraindicated for your condition, choose the bath options that are okay for you to use. Your current practitioner may be very open to your efforts to heal through a program such as GAPS. If not, several lists of health practitioners familiar with GAPS are offered through the *Support for You* page at GAPSguide.com.

4. Take note of symptoms you are currently experiencing. Write them down or consider taking "before" photos or videos of skin, behaviours, etc. These records may prove critical to your journey. Note every ache, pain, and frustration. Does your menstrual cycle bring exhaustion? Do you wake throughout the night? Without intervention, do you have a bowel movement

only once every few days? Do you find yourself frequently snapping at your spouse? Once you've jotted down your initial thoughts, fold your list under the back cover of this book. As you think of or notice more issues, add those to your list.

5. Do not try to change your eating yet. There is much to do first. Baby steps!

6. Begin to gather the necessary supplies, as listed in the *Program Tools* section of this Guide (for additional shopping tips, see also this Guide's section *Practical Considerations: GAPS on a Budget*).

7. Continue eating your normal diet.

8. Access cooking fat. If you are comfortable doing so, you can render your own fat at home. Instructions are offered in this Guide's *Recipes: More Essentials* section. If you are not up for rendering your own fat yet, phone four natural/health food stores, butchers, or farms and ask them whether they have or can get in fat rendered from grass-fed, organic animals. Any fat will do, but duck fat is especially versatile. When you find a source, order at least 1 litre (1 quart). If you cannot find a local source, try shopping online. Simply do an Internet search with a phrase such as "order duck fat online" and several options will come up. As with all tips in this Guide, if after some effort this step feels impossible to complete, skip it and purchase another fat you can tolerate instead (e.g., butter, ghee, or coconut oil). Put the fat in your freezer.

9. Continue eating your normal diet.

10. From this book, or from any of the free recipe resources listed on my website, choose one GAPS recipe and practice preparing it. Feel free to entice yourself or your family with a dessert as a starting point (a simple one to try first is the carrot mousse cake recipe listed in this Guide's *Recipes: More Essentials* section).

11. Continue eating your normal diet.

12. Add a GAPS recipe to your regular diet (even just a dessert) whenever you can.

13. Access broth bones. Phone four natural/health food stores, butchers, or farms, and ask them whether they have or can get in bones from grass-fed, organic animals. When you find a source, order or purchase at least 2 kg (4 lbs) of bones. You can ask the supplier for bones "preferably with a bit of meat on and vertically cut to expose the marrow." If that's not available, that's okay! Any bones will do. Store them in your freezer.

14. Continue eating your normal diet, including a GAPS dish here and there.

15. From your natural food store, buy one container of raw, organic, unrefined apple cider vinegar. Ask a staff person to show you where it is.

16. Continue eating your normal diet, including a GAPS dish here and there.

17. Take one or more soup bones out of the freezer. Put the bone(s) into a bowl large enough to contain it and catch any drippings. Put the bowl of bone in the fridge and let thaw 24–48 hours.

18. Continue eating your normal diet.

19. From this Guide's *Recipes: More Essentials* section, use a bone (with or without meat on it) to make a broth. Use the *Meat Broth* recipe, simmering for just one to three hours.

20. Continue eating your normal diet, adding broth to soups or to veggie dishes, and enjoying the occasional GAPS dish or dessert.

21. From this Guide's *Recipes: Soups for Intro* section, make one soup.

22. Continue eating your normal diet, adding broth, soups, or other GAPS dishes and desserts.

23. Once or twice a week, make a GAPS soup. Use one of the recipes from within this Guide or one from any of the free recipe sources linked to from GAPSguide.com.

24. With the addition of soups and any other GAPS dishes (including desserts), continue eating your normal diet. Don't worry if you or your kids don't crave the soups yet. Don't force it. Intro, coming soon enough, will shift each family member's tastes quite quickly. For now, eat what you enjoy, put the rest into containers with a list of ingredients attached to each, and freeze them.

25. Start using your new source of quality fat (preferably from the inside of any animal) for your general cooking, reheating, and baking. If your body struggles with fat, start with a very small amount—even 5 mL (1 teaspoon)—and work up. See also this Guide's section *Health Issues: Fat Malabsorption.*

26. Other than the broth, soups, fat, and any other GAPS dishes you enjoy, continue eating your normal diet.

27. Phone four stores, starting with natural/health food stores, and ask them whether they have or can get in meat from grass-fed, organic (preferably pastured) animals. When you find a source, order or purchase a whole chicken (if you do not tolerate or enjoy chicken, any other meat will do equally well). Put it in the freezer.

28. Take your chicken (or other meat) out of the freezer. Put it in a bowl large enough to contain it and catch any drippings. Put it in the fridge and let thaw 24 hours. After 24 hours, remove any plastics from inside and outside of the

chicken. Put the chicken into a pot. Cover with water. Bring to a boil and then simmer for two to three hours. When finished, let the pot cool. Remove the chicken and put it into a bowl. Put the chicken and the broth, separately, into the fridge. Within 24 hours, move to the next step.

29. When the broth has cooled, you may or may not find a thick layer of fat on top or that all of the liquid has gelled. Any way is fine. Complete the following steps (this may take a good hour the first time):

- Place the chicken onto a clean surface.

- Remove the major pieces of meat and put them into one bowl.

- Put all the other soft stuff (e.g., skin and fat) into another bowl. Add a bit of meat and some salt to this bowl and blend. Put this mixture into a freezer container labelled "pâté" and refrigerate or freeze it.

- Ladle the broth into small, 500–750 mL (2–3 cup) containers for freezing. Place one container in the fridge and the rest in the freezer.

- Portion most of the meat into small freezer containers and freeze all except one day's worth of meat, which will go into the fridge.

30. Add meat or pâté to your next soup or other meal.

31. From this point forward, continue choosing and preparing various GAPS recipes. Aim for one GAPS meal per day. Other than those meals, continue eating your normal diet.

32. Increase to two GAPS meals per day on as many days as you can manage. Other than those meals, continue eating your normal diet.

FOOD AND ENTERTAINMENT

This point in your progress is a good time to consider a key piece that will make a world of difference in doing GAPS: shifting our perception from "food as entertainment" to "food as fuel." When we make this shift, our lives are transformed. Indeed, success in GAPS will depend very much on finding diversion, joy, and stimulation in activities that are not centred on food. These can include reading, watching movies, playing, conversing, meditating, dancing, listening to music, drawing, hiking, playing cards, playing an instrument, and so on. Unless the entertainment needs that had previously been met by food are replaced with new and equally wonderful diversions, children and adults alike will struggle with a program like GAPS. We can definitely find much sensory pleasure in the rich and diverse meals available within GAPS, as well as continue to enjoy the social and celebratory aspects of birthday parties, potlucks, Halloween, and other food-focused events. We'll simply shift away from food being a primary form of entertainment.

33. When you are consistently eating two GAPS meals per day, increase to three GAPS meals per day as many days as you can manage.

34. Review the *Fermented Fish* recipe offered in this Guide. For this recipe, buy fish that has been commercially frozen for at least two weeks (to kill parasites), then store it in your own freezer.

35. When you are consistently eating three GAPS meals per day, add GAPS-friendly snacks.

36. Make a jar of fermented vegetables. It is super easy to make and we won't make you eat it if you don't want to! For now, just put the ingredients in a jar and set the jar anywhere that is approximately 21°C–24°C (70°F–75°F).

37. If you are opting to start the supplements early in your program, purchase them now (delivery may take up to two weeks). For information on selecting and ordering, review the *Supplementation* section of this Guide.

38. Connect with a support option (live, online, or phone). Many people at this stage of transition won't necessarily feel the need for additional help yet, but it is still important to complete this step at this stage. It can take time to connect with a group, learn how an online group works, have your posts taken off moderation, or find a suitable phone buddy. Thus, it will benefit you greatly to choose and connect with a support option before starting Intro or Full GAPS, and before you run into challenges. For options, go to GAPSguide.com and click on the *Support for You* page. There you will find a list of support options and blogs to consider and choose from. Note: Do not try to memorize everything you read within a blog or forum, or even to understand everything. The key at this stage is to know that warm, loving, nurturing support exists and that there is a place to ask questions as they come up!

39. From the list of health practitioners linked to from the *Support for You* page at GAPSguide.com, narrow down which practitioners you might like to consult with if needed.

40. Set a monthly reminder in your electronic calendar to check both Dr. Campbell-McBride's FAQ document and the *Book Updates* page on GAPSguide.com. (Any new information that I learn, or any corrections to the contents of this edition, will be posted to the *Book Updates* page, so please be sure to check it regularly.)

41. Once your diet is 100% GAPS, continue to enjoy Full GAPS for several weeks or months. During this period, begin considering and implementing some of the other tips in this Guide (e.g., shopping for a child-friendly

enema, reducing clutter, or planning a GAPS-friendly celebration). If you know, or suspect, that you have a sensitivity to a given food or food group, this is a perfect time to rotate it out (See the *Food Issues: Food Sensitivities/Allergies* section of this Guide). Continue to enjoy Full GAPS until you feel ready to start Intro. To determine your ready point, please review the following material.

Approaching Intensive Healing

"Stage 2 includes raw yolk added to soup; can I do a whole, soft-boiled egg instead?" • *"I really believe in raw foods; can't I start those earlier?"* • *"I just don't want to do my lunches without bread; would it really be a problem if I started it now? I promise I'd use coconut flour!"* • *"I know other people might need to start with a smaller amount of probiotic, but I've been eating WAPF for two years, so I'm sure I can handle two capsules of a probiotic right off the bat."* • *"A daily dose of selenium has been so helpful to me. Do I really need to exclude it from my Intro program?"*

At some point in GAPS' Intro, most of us will bump full force into our own psychological barriers. Food concepts learned pre-GAPS may strongly conflict with what GAPS is presenting, and 30 years of established eating habits lead us to believe we "cannot" eat soup for breakfast or that we "must" have a banana right now! We can feel frustrated, resentful, or even angry. I know this all too well! I came to GAPS absolutely repulsed by soup, bananas, eggs, gelatin, leftovers, and freshly cooked food (I had been becoming increasingly phobic about any food not presented in a sealed package). Upon starting the program, I found that I also couldn't stand the taste of SCD yogurt or fermented cod liver oil and I was terrified of my first batch of home-fermented vegetables. Finally, the first time I tried to eat meat after 22 years of vegetarianism, I burst into tears of grief!

At this point in our journey, we often ask GAPS veterans for permission or support to do something other than the GAPS Intro progression as set out. We bargain: "What if I jump ahead, but then have two detox baths right after?" We threaten: "If someone doesn't say I can have a handful of dates today, I'm quitting!" (Indeed, how many times did I threaten to quit if someone didn't tell me "by today" how to get the yogurt right, or how I could do this as a vegetarian?) Here are some of my thoughts:

Each person's body is theirs to do with as they wish. Everything you ingest, and the timing and order of ingestion, is your choice. I support and celebrate that. GAPS is presented, but it is never forced. None of us is in your home demanding that you do anything in a specific way. You are truly free to "do GAPS" or to simply practice some of the concepts from GAPS or to do something else altogether. If you choose to do GAPS, which means doing it as presented, there are a whole bunch of us available to support you because we know how to help you when you're doing GAPS.

I present GAPS because I believe GAPS to be an excellent approach to healing. I have no attachment to whether people do it or do not do it, but I can present only what GAPS is. If folks choose to take any other path, I am not able to provide peer support only because I can't speak to any of the variables that may come up with any other path—even if you feel it is "very close to GAPS" or "GAPS with just a few changes."

What we introduce, in what order, and when, is explicitly detailed in the list of GAPS-recommended foods and in the Intro progression. If you choose to do something different than that which is set out, that is your prerogative. However, in this case the GAPS community can't speak to how well or quickly your healing will progress, what challenges may arise, or how to address those challenges.

If you face difficulties and have done something other than that which is set out, I will always recommend you go back to "square one" and start again following the directions exactly. When a person follows the GAPS directions exactly and faces a challenge, we can better help narrow down the issue.

There is a reason for the Intro progression (and all other details of GAPS). Dr. Campbell-McBride is a very kind and loving doctor who would not ask us to undertake anything that is more challenging than absolutely necessary. Dr. Campbell-McBride has set out steps based on many hours of clinical research, sound study, and a desire to see each of us heal as efficiently as possible. If it worked to do things any other way, she would let us know. What is set out is the best (and full range of) information we currently have.

Some people do choose to veer from the directions and some of these people still experience success. This is awesome and helps inform research and the future of GAPS. If you decide to veer, you may still see success and you should feel free to share those details with others. However, GAPS veterans will continue teaching what they know to be tried and true for many.

The GAPS community is unique among dietary ones in that it does not demand perfection. If you choose to do something other than presented, you are supported in speaking freely in the GAPS support forums about that. Just be aware that folks—myself included—generally won't have the resources to discuss the potential outcomes of any given variation proposed.

All of us come to GAPS having learned and practiced something different in the past (otherwise we wouldn't be here now). We have been told that meat is hard to digest, that the body prefers veggies raw, and that grains are crucial to the human diet. Also, until one's body heals to some degree, one's intuition tends to be off. Finally, before we see results, we have no solid reason to believe in a "bizarre new diet." For all of these reasons, we're strongly tempted to do our own thing: to tweak, to play, to veer, to experiment. I believe that if we are going to do GAPS, we need to trust Dr. Campbell-McBride's recommendations long enough to give it a good go, and give it a chance to show results. This is not to say you should override your own intuition or the recommendations of your health practitioner, but rather that we can honour these while simultaneously checking in with our own mental (as opposed to intuitive) barriers and addressing those. The good news is that when the results come, it becomes infinitely easier to simply follow the directions! Today, I am very grateful that I chose to override my original preferences and ideas in order to commit to GAPS as presented.

Regarding how to approach supplements, I recommend:

- Slowly weaning off supplements *not required for life or limb* before starting Intro;
- Beginning GAPS with just food;
- Only after a range of food has been reintroduced, begin adding GAPS-recommended bottled foods such as cod liver oil, a commercial probiotic, fish oil, and nut/seed oil; and
- Only after several months of healing or under the guidance of a GAPS-knowledgeable practitioner, including additional elements as your body indicates need.

There are multiple reasons to ingest only what is necessary during the early stages of healing. Benefits include:

1. An opportunity to see what your body experiences and "says."
2. An opportunity to witness the impact of and healing effects of whole foods.
3. An opportunity to learn how to adjust diet to relieve symptoms and promote healing.
4. Avoidance of any gut aggravation imposed by extra ingredients commonly found in supplements.
5. Elimination of unnecessary expense, reserving funds for food and other critical resources.

The aspect of "including additional elements as your body indicates need" must be recognized. Supplements and medications can indeed be useful adjuncts to a powerful healing protocol. Vitamin C can help relieve constipation;

magnesium can do likewise while also eliminating leg cramps and promoting sleep. People with an illness as severe as Crohn's disease or adrenal burnout may require medication or supplementation during the initial part of their journey. For more information, see the sections *Supplementation* and *Health Issues: Medication.*

Again, GAPS and similar healing programs present a basic protocol, with *most* recommendations bringing excellent results to *most* people. There are strong advantages to following it "as is." However, once you have a few months of progress under your belt, or earlier if extreme need dictates, feel free to explore any adjunct approaches that may encourage and assist your body's healing (some do this on their own; some with the assistance of a health practitioner familiar with GAPS). The key is to allow your body and mind opportunity to experience and observe the effects of a simple, food-based program rather than to leap from one symptom-specific remedy to another. In other words, a remedy should be a minor adjunct to a program that is well thought out, longer term, deeply nourishing, free from gut aggravators (if possible), and actively healing—all of which GAPS is.

Foundations for Healing

Two key factors that can make or break your healing journey are *rest* and *trust*.

The process of healing demands a lot of energy. Healing (and also hormonal support) is directly dependent on rest. Support your body to complete the process. Don't wait until your health becomes so frail that you are incapacitated and unable to work and exercise; invest a relatively short period of your life now to allow for healing. Too many of us (me included) became so debilitated through our pre-GAPS diet that we became unable to work, do self-care, or exercise for several months or even years. Although it can be painful financially to take some time off, it is far cheaper in the long run to do so in commitment to healing rather than to push your body to the point of incapacitation. Especially for your first time on Intro, and unless you intuit that you would be well-served by distractions, try to arrange one to six weeks off of some or all of your regular activities. During the first days, you may feel incredibly lethargic. During your subsequent weeks on Intro, you can expect to experience various changes in the body (e.g., lethargy with every new round of die-off). You will need more time to shop, cook, journal, research, access online support, sleep, rest, and/or take detox baths. In response to both the digestive rest and the inclusion of dense nutrition, your body will want to heal. When the conflicting activities of rushing, working, exercising, schooling, or unceasing care of children are imposed on the more essential physical processes, we may find ourselves struggling deeply. For all of these reasons, reducing your overall activity level can be a great gift to your body and may make all the difference in healing, especially in those with adrenal issues, for example. A trip to the park, reading, or a couple of hours of work on a light project can provide essential distraction, but trying to press through your usual life while implementing an intense healing effort can backfire. Take time off work, put your fitness membership on temporary hold, arrange extra childcare, and so on.

One of the strongest commitments I make to my son besides nutrition is rest. He is ensured lots of downtime and has a bedtime as early as 6:30 PM depending on the time of year, his activities that day, and his level of energy versus fatigue. Although an early bedtime means skipping evening events, the benefits of a long rest—and waking only when his body (as opposed to an alarm) triggers him to— are obvious in him. I have seen the lives of other children, too, change dramatically when their parents accommodate a bedtime far earlier than today's norm. For more information regarding rest, please see this Guide's section *Health Issues: Exercise.*

A second foundation for healing is trust. This quality is manifested in our willingness to follow the program, rest when our body is tired, eat as frequently as the body indicates need, prioritize healing over the financial gains achieved through excess work, increase our fats and/or carbohydrates when our body requests this, and incorporate adjunct healing protocols as our intuition urges us.

In this Guide, I set out very specific steps. I do so because so many people feel lost without such and crave a starting point. The process presented in this Guide has been developed on the basis of many people's experiences, so they work well for most people. However, no program or Guide can know your body's needs as well as your own body can. If any suggestion within this Guide is not a good fit for you, please do what your body needs you to do.

An additional aspect of trusting the body involves the order of healing. Although you may desire a given symptom to resolve immediately, it is the body that decides in which order and within which timeframe symptoms will heal. We can certainly support the body's movement toward health, but we cannot override its decisions about what heals first or how soon any given symptom resolves. The order and timing for each symptom's resolution is different for everyone.

"What if I cheat on the diet?" On the one hand, I recommend that a person "aim for 100% adherence in order to achieve 95%." On the other hand, I note that in the process of recovering our health, there is no judge, thus there cannot really be "cheating." Over the course of healing, each of us will at some points either accidentally or consciously ingest a food not on the recommended list. Those of us who are particularly curious or stubborn may actually require the occasional experiment in order to truly grasp the tremendous power of food! Use the error or experiment as an opportunity to observe your body's reactions. In the meantime, eating some fermented foods may help the body process the undesirable item. Also, when the error is contained to one meal, Dr. Campbell-McBride suggests in her FAQ document that an adult take betaine HCL with pepsin (1–4 capsules depending on the size of the meal) and 10–15 minutes later take 2–5 capsules of a "full pancreatic formula." In the case of a strong reaction, a detox bath, a dose of activated charcoal, and/or a few days on Stage 1 before picking up where you left off, may help. If the experiment has gone on a little too long, consider restarting with Intro, running fairly quickly through the Stages until you are back at your optimal menu. In short, simply get back on track as soon as possible. Folks recovering from addiction to heroin or alcohol who relapse will summon much courage and faith in order to start over on any given day. Let this inspire us to do likewise!

Transitional Discomfort in Healing

In early healing, the body goes through many changes. Many of the changes will be welcomed: we will feel clearer, lighter, and happier. We will begin to laugh again. Many of us will sing more often. Confidence will rise, thoughts will be clearer, joy will bubble up. We will experience a calm, peaceful, thoughtful response to issues that previously triggered anger. In adults, libido will balance, such that an uncomfortable hypersexuality is mellowed or an abated sex drive is reignited. Sleep will deepen. Initially, though, we may not feel these positive effects, but rather significant discomfort! Additionally, over the long-term course of healing, the body will regularly commit to deeper healing, at which points discomfort will again be experienced. Generally, each round of intensive healing will be less uncomfortable. Also, as we become more experienced in how to care for our bodies, remedying each round of discomfort will be faster and easier.

As it heals, the body begins to trust that it will get what it needs to sustain optimal health. Thus, it begins to reprioritize its goal from mere survival to vigorous health. In this process, mineral composition shifts, microbes that thrive only in an undernourished system begin to die-off, bacteria which support the transmission of minerals to all parts of the body reclaim their territory, fuel sources transition, various elements in healing foods begin their "clean up" activities, and toxins are released from tissue and transported through the body for release. These changes are exciting, significant, and—in most people—deeply felt. Three major sources of discomfort associated with these changes are (1) "detox" (also known as the Herxheimer reaction or die-off), (2) toxic backlog, and (3) ketosis.

Detox, Die-Off, and Toxic Backlog

As the body's healing systems are rejuvenated, and detoxifying substances are introduced to the body, toxins are naturally released from their storage sites and transported through the body for release through urine, stool, bile, and sweat. Also, when pathogenic microbes die off, they release toxins. During the period in which toxins are freed from tissue or are temporarily produced, but have not yet been removed from the body, you will experience discomfort. This discomfort is temporary and usually lasts anywhere from a few hours to a few days, but it can persist for up to several weeks (especially when the steps presented within this Guide are disregarded, or when a person comes to the program in a deeply ill state). To reduce the intensity and duration of any discomfort, it is essential to remove toxins efficiently.

Symptoms of die-off and/or toxic backlog can include: bloating, diarrhea, dizziness, pain, soreness, fatigue, weakness, constipation, sneezing, nausea, vomiting, headache, muscle aches, reflux, depression, sleep disturbances (including any degree of insomnia), renewal of self-stimulation (e.g., flapping, rocking, and vocalizations), lethargy, pallor, mood swings, confusion or "brain fog," irritability, whining, tantrums, and other behavioural difficulties, rashes, anger, and/or an increase in any symptom that brought you to the diet. Although I have emphasized some of these in the section *What to Expect in Intro*, these can also occur upon removing a single problematic food from your diet, at any point in your transition to GAPS, or at any point within the two-year program of healing. Forewarned is forearmed—there are several ways to reduce the speed of detox, the rate of die-off, and the amount of toxic backlog.

Relief from Transitional Discomfort

- Before going on the Intro diet, slowly wean yourself off foods that are not included on GAPS. Ideally, do this by including progressively more GAPS meals into your diet. The month(s) spent completing the steps under *Preparing for Full GAPS/Intro* are very helpful for this.

- Introduce and increase probiotics and yeast killers very carefully. For example, if using the probiotic Bio-Kult, a child might start on one-tenth of a capsule (or less) with the dosage slowly increased from there, increasing by perhaps another one-tenth of a capsule just once every week or two (see this Guide's section *Supplementation: Probiotics*). Early in my healing, I glibly increased my probiotic from one capsule to two and I experienced far more die-off than I wanted to. Cutting back helped. Also early in the program, I started the yeast-reducing probiotic, *Saccharomyces boulardii (S. boulardii)*, at full dosage and my dormant OCD rose up with a vengeance. A capsule of activated charcoal relieved this, but the lesson stayed with me. When I reintroduced *S. boulardii* a few months later, I eased into it without any problems. I cannot emphasize enough the importance of going "low and slow" with all healing elements, including diet, probiotics, and antifungals.

- Ensure a minimum of one to three bowel movements per day.

- Drink lots of water and/or replenishing drinks (see *Recipes: More Essentials*).

- Drink lots of broth and/or meat stock.

- Take one to three detox baths daily.

- Get lots of rest (e.g, watch gentle, inspiring DVDs or read positive, encouraging books).

- Enjoy very gentle exercise, such as a slow walk in fresh air.

- Take a magnesium supplement. This is helpful to many people in early healing to address constipation and also to relieve anxiety, panic attacks, depression, pain, muscle aches, insomnia, headaches, stress, restless leg syndrome, and cramping. Epsom salts are a source of magnesium; soaking in an Epsom salt bath can provide excellent results. A popular magnesium supplement used by many GAPSters is Magnesium Citrate Powder by Natural Calm Canada (www.naturalcalm.ca). Your health practitioner or health food store (local or online) can direct you to other options or one balanced with complementary minerals for longer term use. As your range of food increases, you will be able to access increasing amounts of magnesium—with the same effects—through GAPS foods and juices.

- Take vitamin C to bowel tolerance (i.e., increasing the dose until stools are loose, then continuing to use the dose immediately previous to that one).

- Incorporate a clay remedy, as recommended by your health practitioner or local health food store.

- If transitional discomfort is very bothersome, a dose of activated charcoal may be very helpful.
- Consider the following additional information regarding ketosis and carbohydrates.

People often read the above tips, ignore them, leap into the program, experience terrible discomfort, and then post to GAPSguide.com asking what they should do. The best approach is to move gently through the program, as presented in this Guide, being as kind to yourself as possible by applying the above tips from the start.

Ketosis and Carbohydrates

Questions about carbohydrates and ketosis are often asked within the GAPS community. Here I explore both of these topics, their relationship to each other, and the options available to those doing GAPS.

First, to directly address a common misconception, the diet aspect of GAPS is based on the Specific Carbohydrate Diet (SCD), not a low-carbohydrate diet. The SCD is concerned with the type of carbohydrate; it does not ask one to restrict the amount. Although GAPS is not a low-carbohydrate program specifically, it is often lower in both total carbohydrates and "net" carbohydrates (e.g., carbohydrate count minus total fibre count) than a conventional diet is. This may trigger concern in some people.

Early in GAPS, I calculated my carbohydrates. I was getting approximately 200 grams per day, or ten times the amount suggested for a low-carb diet. On many days, over 150 grams (approximately 75%) of my carbs were coming from the copious vegetables I was eating. According to *SELF* Nutrition Data (www.nutritiondata.com), my carb data then was:

Food	Carbs (grams)
Well-cooked veggies (approximately 4 litres or 15 cups per day, measured raw, in stew)	100–120
Juiced veggies	38
Cashew butter (125 mL or ½ cup on a big day)	33
Honey (average 5 mL per day, taken as 15 mL every 2–3 days)	9
Avocado (½)	8
Ghee	0
Meats	0
TOTAL:	**188–208**

As I progressed through Intro, the volume of food I was eating reduced, but the carbohydrate count remained about the same. The carbohydrates found in the enormous amounts of vegetables I initially started out eating were easily replaced by the eventual incorporation of fruit and an increase in nuts.

Many people experience significant healing by severely reducing or eliminating carbohydrates for a short or long period of time (as I did, to my great benefit, a few weeks before the above data was collected). For many people, doing so resolves seizures, reduces unhealthy weight, and/or eliminates cravings for sweets and grains. In reducing one's carbohydrate intake, the body adapts to a different source of fuel. Among other benefits, this often allows chronically underweight people to finally bring their weight up to desired levels (after a brief period of loss). Indeed, some people find that a diet free of carbohydrates—and based entirely on animal sources—is what supports their optimal health.

What about ketosis? Ketosis[1] occurs when the body no longer has access to glucose (from carbohydrates) and transitions to sourcing its energy, indirectly, from fat. While every person (whether doing GAPS or not) experiences degrees of ketosis over the course of any given day or week, people in the early stages of GAPS may experience a more sustained ketosis than otherwise occurs throughout any period on a conventional diet. The transitioning of fuel sources can result in some discomfort; this usually lasts less than a week. Signs that the body is transitioning its fuel source may include reduced appetite, brain fog, fatigue, dehydration, and constipation. Some people believe consistent ketosis is dangerous; some believe it is benign. If you have any concerns, consult with a health practitioner familiar with a program like GAPS.

For most people, any discomfort associated with sustained ketosis will resolve within the first week of Intro. Many of the tips presented under *Relief from Transitional Discomfort* will help. A replenishing drink can be especially helpful — even one without a source of carbohydrates (e.g., honey).

Although there are specific benefits to reducing carbohydrates and even to going into a strong degree of ketosis, if one finds the transitional discomfort unbearable or for any other reason prefers to keep their carbohydrate count up, doing so is an option. Some sources suggest that as few as 35 grams of carbohydrates per day will keep a person out of ketosis. Even in Stage 1 of GAPS, more than this is easy to achieve: if a person adds 5 mL (1 teaspoon) of honey to each of three cups of tea or replenishing drink, and enjoys 250 mL (1 cup) of butternut squash, and a soup containing 250 mL (1 cup) of carrots and 250 mL (1 cup) of onions, she has already taken in approximately 73 grams of

---

[1] Ketosis is not to be confused with ketoacidosis, which can be life-threatening to those with Type 1 diabetes.

carbohydrates. Add another cup of carrots and another cup of onions in a hearty soup and she will have ingested approximately 105 grams of carbohydrates. (Note that the minimum number of grams of carbohydrates needed to keep a person out of ketosis, or at optimal health and energy levels long term, is different for everyone. Also, the number can change based on a person's health history, age, size, gender, level of activity, and so on.)

Some people do choose to avoid the discomfort of ketosis by ensuring that even their earliest days of Intro include large amounts of higher carbohydrate GAPS vegetables. Although avoiding transitional discomfort may help a person stick with the program, it should be noted that in some people this approach can delay healing and perpetuate cravings for sweet foods. I recommend simply being prepared for some degree of discomfort and relying on the tips for relieving transitional discomfort.

If you have any concerns or questions about ketosis, or about your own optimal carbohydrate count or needs at any given point in your GAPS program, please consult with a health practitioner familiar with GAPS.

CHAPTER 6

MONTHS 4–6: GAPS INTRO PROGRESSION

Again, you may opt for a slightly different timeline than this book presents, and that's fine. If you have spent at least two months preparing for the program, with at least the final week or two of that time enjoying Full GAPS, you might at this point consider beginning GAPS' Intro protocol, an intensive healing phase of the program.

When to do Intro

Our timing can make or break our success with Intro. Many people have jumped in at a random time, only to feel the need to quit shortly thereafter. Before starting Intro, it is worth considering several factors:

1. **Do you have everything you need?** Have you connected with sources for ingredients? Have you practiced some of the recipes, especially the basics (e.g., broth, soup, and fermented vegetables)? Have you weaned yourself from processed foods? Have you begun to change the focus of your family activities so that they are not centred around food? If you answered "no" to any of these questions, I strongly recommend starting at the beginning of the section *Months 1–3: Preparing for Full GAPS/Intro* before proceeding to Intro.

2. **What's happening around you?** Hot weather, major holidays, religious events, cultural festivities, the start of the school year, and intense work demands can challenge your success in Intro. Many people prefer to start the Intro protocol during a cooler season—making the temptation of garden-fresh veggies moot, and fats and hot soups far more desirable—and away from any major family or cultural events, such as the start of a new school year, an annual visit from in-laws, Ramadan, birthday parties, Easter, Halloween, or Christmas. For example, for some people in Canada or the United States, one ideal time to start might be New Year's Day, January 1st. Scheduling Intro for an ideal time in your personal calendar will allow you to honour a need to eat every hour or so, focus on healing without feeling deprived of traditions, develop a preference for GAPS food well before a sweets-centred event occurs, stay home during intense die-off, fully enjoy a visit from rarely seen friends, and more fully support short-term houseguests. Consider a six-week period of time when the weather is not hot in your area, there is not an abundance of tempting garden-fresh vegetables available, there are not any major food-centred events or holidays, and there are not any major work- or family-related priorities.

3. **Do you have children?** If yes, you may want to do Intro before walking them through it. This will give you much more physical and emotional strength to support them through the process. It will also help you to understand what is happening inside your children physically and emotionally as they move through the different stages. Some families even choose to put each child on Intro one at a time, with the rest of the family eating beyond that stage, so that only one is going through healing crisis at a time and the rest are available to provide support. (In this scenario, I urge all other members of the family to eat more advanced foods only out of sight of the person on Intro.)

4. **Is your need urgent?** Regardless of any of the above, you may decide that healing is more important than some other aspects of life, and choose to start as soon as you are sufficiently prepared for it. My son and I started Intro during a very hot month in a semi-arid region without so much as air-conditioning! For us, healing was more important than waiting for cool weather. At least that month was well away from any birthday or the beginning of school!

How Long Does Intro Last?

The complete Intro progression involves six stages. Most people move through the full six stages of the Intro progression in about six weeks. Each person will spend a different amount of time on each introduction or stage, each moving slower through some and faster through others. A few people will stay on an early stage for several weeks or months, but this is relatively rare. Pacing and when to move forward is discussed later in this chapter.

Who Should do Intro and Why?

GAPS' Intro is very helpful to most people, regardless of symptoms or nutritional background. Some people have skipped Intro because they did not know about it, or on another's advice that it was not necessary, or out of fear of experiencing die-off, or out of reluctance to give up favourite foods even for a short time. Many who initially thought that they did not need Intro have reported that their greatest gains were achieved by finally doing it. Indeed, the six-stage progression of Intro provides many benefits, such as:

- Quickly changing gut flora for fast, whole-body (including mind and behavioural) results.
- Infusing our body with nutrition, by removing barriers to digestion and including optimal foods.

- Allowing us to create new food habits one step at a time.

- Helping identify food intolerances previously unrecognized.

- Helping us get past food aversions and refusals, and expanding our ability to take in a wider range of foods.

- Helping us establish or re-establish fundamental aspects of GAPS (e.g., broths or ferments).

- Helping us appreciate the incredible variety within Full GAPS.

- Reducing or eliminating sugar cravings, leaving us with more balanced requirements for sweetness.

- Helping us learn about stool types, our bodies' signals, and our bodies' needs.

- Allowing us to experience how simple meal preparation can actually be.

- Freeing our time for other healing activities, such as resting, going for walks, or spending time with friends.

- Supporting a speedy recovery from illness or stress.

- Encouraging us to learn food preparations we might not have tried otherwise.

All that gained within just six weeks of your life!

Who Should Skip Intro

Women who are either pregnant or breast-feeding are advised to delay Intro until after these life stages have passed. For more information, please see the section *Special Considerations: GAPS through Life's Stages.*

What to Expect in Intro

In preparing for or eating Full GAPS, you may have experienced changes in your body (some people will have experienced changes even upon removing a single food, such as wheat). Whether or not this was true for you, the Intro progression will almost definitely trigger a range of experiences. Many of these changes will be welcomed (e.g., increased energy, balanced weight, clearer skin, and better mood); others may cause concern. The most common of these temporary changes include constipation, extreme lethargy, pallor, irritability, total loss of appetite, dramatic increase in hunger, sadness, flu-like symptoms, aches, heartburn, skin eruptions, and insomnia. Children, especially, may experience a total loss of appetite, extreme lethargy, and vomiting. For most people, the worst of the transition occurs between Day 1 and Day 5, then resolves. Lighter versions of this discomfort may recur at various intervals throughout the two-year program (this is true regardless of changes or lack of changes to one's program).

Some or all of these changes will be due to die-off. Some changes may be attributed to ketosis, discussed earlier. Whether due to die-off or ketosis, you can expect to feel any or all of the following:

- **Aches:** Ouchy, pinging, I-feel-like-I-just-ran-a-marathon-without-training-first aches. These can appear in random parts of the body or all over. During die-off, when I'm climbing out of the bathtub or walking, I have an experience in my muscles akin to when I'm lifting weights. The sensation makes me think of wading through quicksand. It's intense! (At these points, my breathing is also somewhat laboured.)

- **Appetite changes:** The Intro food is very digestible, plus your body will be using food to fuel tremendous changes, so you will likely feel ravenous. Conversely, it is common for children to refuse all foods for the first four to five days. Adults, too, may experience a reduced appetite. After this initial stage, expect to be absolutely ravenous for about six weeks before your appetite normalizes. You may need to eat immediately upon waking, and every 60 to 90 minutes for the rest of the day, and then again right before bed. Let your body guide you, eating as it requests—neither more nor less often. Unless you cannot tolerate it, include lots of fat (e.g., animal fat, animal skin, or ghee) in your cooking and add more to the finished meal; the fats will steady your blood sugar, give you energy, and promote overall healing. While ensuring their (very real) hunger is satiated, prepare to also distract children throughout this adjustment period with movies, fun, stories, and outings—simply fill insulated food containers with soup, stew, etc., and head out! This is an intensive healing period; your body will need all the nourishment it is requesting. Fear not! I promise you your appetite will mellow again.

- **Bad breath:** It is common for a person's breath to start smelling "off" in an odd way. For many, the smell is akin to garlic, regardless of whether a person is ingesting garlic or not. In some, it is worse.

- **Body odour:** As we release toxins, our body odour can become intense. Some things that help include die-off relief baths, spraying your armpits with a solution of apple cider vinegar mixed with water while showering, and sprinkling baking soda on the smelly parts. Feel free to use a salt deodorant.

REMEMBER

We may feel quite self-conscious for the first while, but it will be worth it!

- **Boredom:** During Intro, we realize how much we use food (i.e., shopping, planning, cooking, and eating) as entertainment. In the simplicity of Intro, we can find ourselves with a lot of time (possibly in combination with reduced energy), and may end up feeling very bored. Have gentle, non-food activities ready, such as meditation, reading, movies, knitting, board games, and so on.

- **Cold or flu symptoms:** Many people report that cold or flu-like symptoms appear during Intro. There are several theories for this, the primary one being that the body is relieving itself of stored viruses.

- **Confusion or overwhelm:** Despite the steps being laid out in this Guide as clearly as I could manage, many people will still feel overwhelmed or confused. This is sometimes a result of feeling we should do things in ways other than laid out. If this is the case for you, consider following the steps as written, one step at a time—no changes—adding a new food, supplement, or cooking style every four days or so. Simple as that. Again, starting at the beginning of the *Months 1–3: Preparing for Full GAPS/Intro* section can help a lot!

- **Cravings:** For tips on addressing these, please see this Guide's section *Health Issues: Cravings and Hunger.*

- **Emotional issues:** These can appear as sadness, depression, fear, nostalgia, painful memories, frustration, nightmares, anger, or resentment about any aspect of the program. Although no one enjoys these states, try not to fear them. The process of healing will naturally include the resurfacing, and subsequent resolution of, emotional issues. Besides applying the standard self-care tools such as die-off management, be prepared to implement other supports, such as inspiring movies, conversations with friends, meditation, prayer, eye movement desensitization and reprocessing (EMDR), Emotional Freedom Techniques (EFT), art, walks, rest and naps, or counselling. Connecting with other GAPSters via the e-mail or phone lists can make all the difference. These folks will be able to hear you, comfort you, encourage you, and guide you toward more self-care. In a pinch, a crisis line may also be a good resource for talking through any emotional discomfort.

- **Fatigue:** This can be profound. Some people can barely get off the couch for a day or so; others can get up, but cannot walk five blocks. As stated previously, rest is a foundation for healing. Allow for this. Honour your body.

- **Heart rate changes, increase or decrease in blood pressure, palpitations:** Some people note any of these symptoms after drinking broth, taking a detox bath, or eating any histamine-containing food. If the symptom persists, adjust your program (e.g., removing the triggering food, using only the detox bath additives that do not trigger these symptoms, or using only long-fermented vegetables). Dr. Campbell-McBride suggests magnesium for high blood pressure. For more information on these symptoms, see Dr. Campbell-McBride's FAQ document.

- **Increased or resurfaced symptoms:** You may temporarily experience a resurfacing of any historical symptom, or more deeply any of the symptoms that brought you to GAPS. This may present as an ache in a previously broken bone, stimming, acne, tics, eczema, reflux, or anxiety, for example.

- **Nausea:** Any one or more of the following may help feelings of nausea: eating a small, fat-and-protein meal upon waking and then every hour or so throughout the day until right before bed; sipping a replenishing drink—especially an electrolyte drink—throughout the day; sipping ginger tea; taking a die-off relief bath; having a bowel movement; taking a gentle walk in the fresh air; and taking a nap.

- **Reflux:** Many people come to GAPS to resolve the symptoms of reflux, which can be triggered by low stomach acid levels. Ironically, this symptom may worsen initially on Intro, or may become a problem for the first time. Please see the tips in this Guide's section *Health Issues: Heartburn, Reflux, and Indigestion.*

- **Shopping and cooking:** Be prepared to shop and cook a lot during the first four to six weeks. In the very early stages, expect to restock your fridge every one to three days.

- **Skin changes:** A person may appear pale for a few days. Also, temporary skin eruptions (e.g., rashes, pimples, warts, cold sores, and eczema) are quite common as the body releases toxins and stored viruses.

- **Sleep changes:** You may find yourself needing to go to bed earlier. Conversely, insomnia in any of its forms may become an issue.

- **Stool changes:** For several months after starting Intro, let go of any expectations you may have about what stool "should be" like. Regardless of what you do or don't do, your stool may be "all over the map" for some time. In the first few months, it may be on various days: smelly, non-existent, black, small, tar-like, mucousy, fluffy, green, floating, grey, sinking, or containing visible pieces of food—you name it. Unless you experience cramping, or a true, potentially dehydrating diarrhea, or see blood from the inside of the bowels (as opposed to small amounts that may result from constipated stool stretching or otherwise irritating the anus), ignore the stool. Simply ensure something comes out daily. For more information, see this Guide's section *Detoxification: Bowel Movements*.

- **Tooth discolouration:** A number of people have experienced a distinct discolouration of their teeth at various points on GAPS (or the SCD and other healing programs). It appears to relate to a shift in bacterial balance within the mouth, and it is possibly related to iron. It often develops in tandem with other die-off symptoms. The grey-to-black hue appears to be inside the tooth, but the colour is actually superficial and will come off with a professional cleaning, if not a home one. I now brush with a Philips Sonicare toothbrush plus random applications of baking soda or any commercial toothpaste; this has prevented further rounds of discolouration. For details of my journey with this symptom, please refer to the GAPSguide.com website. In terms of general oral hygiene not specific to greying, see also this Guide's section *Detoxification: Avoiding Chemicals—Personal Care*.

- **Urination:** Expect lots and lots and lots of it. Urine is one of the avenues through which the body releases toxins. Children may start wetting the bed at night. As with all the issues listed here, this will pass. When bedwetting persists, a sensitivity to a specific food or food element, such as oxalates, may be an issue. In this case, review the information under the *Food Issues: Food Sensitivities/Allergies* section of this Guide. When the level of toxins irritates the bladder lining, you may experience a need to release frequently, or even feel discomfort. In this case, continue applying the tips for preventing or reducing transitional discomfort, plus drink a lot of water and consider cranberry supplementation. If you are at risk of developing a urinary tract infection or other irritation, you can apply homemade kefir or yogurt over the groin area after showering. Again, increased urination on its own is a common effect of deep healing and will pass as the body sorts itself out.

- **Weight changes:** During healing, most people will see a change in their weight. In early Intro, an initial weight loss is often triggered by changing the body's primary fuel source from glucose (from carbohydrates) to fat. A drop in weight can be quite frightening for people whose health issues have already resulted in low weight. However, the initial weight loss is temporary. The healing in general, the inclusion of fats, and/or the increased carbohydrate count as the stages progress allows a balanced weight to be achieved, often for the first time in one's life. Other people, though, want to lose weight or avoid gaining. Again, the initial healing stages will often bring a loss of weight, which can assist in this goal. Note that healing may demand that you allow for pounds temporarily higher than you prefer (but still within a healthy range). Ultimately, weight that you view as too low or too high can be regulated further by healing and, later, by determining one's ideal levels of protein, carbohydrates, exercise, muscle mass, and rest. See the section of this Guide *Progressing Further: Weight adjustments.*

- **Vomiting:** Please see *Nausea.*

Considering the above possibilities, it is no wonder that you may feel discouraged, frustrated, and ready to throw in the towel at points! You may at times feel it is "not worth it." If you hang in there and come out the other side, you will find it was indeed worth doing!

REMEMBER

All of the above is transitional, temporary, and part of the journey to full health. Die-off relief remedies—especially daily bowel movements and daily detox baths—and the slow introduction and increase of probiotics will be critical. Have your plan and supplies ready!

A number of people sail through Intro without a hitch, feeling only good on it, with few or none of the above issues arising. Don't worry: You are healing, too!

Some people complain of other issues, such as hair loss or transitional pain in the abdomen or kidney area. Unfortunately, I don't have information specific to these at the time of this writing (again, for information released subsequent to this book's printing, regularly check the *Book Updates* page at GAPSguide.com as well as Dr. Campbell-McBride's FAQ document). If you are concerned that anything you experience—including any of the issues listed above—may possibly be an indicator of failing health, or you have a concern about a symptom not listed, please contact a health practitioner immediately. One familiar with GAPS may be able to assist you most effectively.

Preparing for Intensive Healing

- Determine your start date.

- Prepare a batch of home-fermented vegetables. The juice of this is introduced early on, and a batch can take up to nine weeks to ferment. If you followed the *Months 1–3: Preparing for Full GAPS/Intro* section, you already have a batch on the go. If you skipped that part, start a batch now. (If you are behind schedule on this, you can look online for a cabbage rejuvelac recipe to use while the vegetables are fermenting.)

- Consider asking others (live or online) to join you on your start date.

- Unless your health practitioner advises otherwise, slowly wean yourself from all supplements and medications not required to preserve life or limb. This includes GAPS oils, probiotics, and other supplements.

- Stock up now on inspiring, cheerful, and uplifting movies, books, and music from your local library.

- Try to arrange one to six weeks off of some of your usual activities, especially if this is your first time on Intro (unless you intuit that you would be well-served by distractions). As noted earlier in this Guide, one of the key aspects to healing is rest, and at points in the early stages of healing you may feel incredibly lethargic. During the weeks of Intro, you can expect to experience various changes in your body, as listed previously, and you will likely also need more time to shop, cook, journal, research, access online support, sleep, rest, and/or take detox baths.

- Arrange extra or stand-by child care.

- Arrange for a friend to pick up groceries for you on Days 2, 4, and 6.

- Consider chopping some veggies. I prefer to chop my 15 cups of Intro vegetables each morning, but others like to have some ready to go. Put each type in a separate bag, and freeze them. Putting each into a separate bag will allow you to test one vegetable at a time and to subsequently exclude any that may be problematic for you. When freezing chopped produce, first lay the pieces on a cookie sheet and put the sheet in the freezer. When they have frozen, move the pieces into a freezer bag. With the pieces frozen individually, you will be able to access just as many as you need at any time.

- Consider preparing some back-up broths. Personally, I find it easiest to just throw a bone into a soup pot every morning, but some people like to have extra broth on hand. Freeze them. Again, make each broth from one animal and label the broths. This will allow you to test—and subsequently exclude, if necessary—any given type.

- Consider doing Intro yourself before walking your child(ren) through it.
- Create a vision board to remind you of the ultimate prize: excellent health!
- Join one of the online support lists, arrange a phone buddy, and/or subscribe to your favourite GAPS blogs. All of these are free. Go to the *Support for You* page at GAPSguide.com to find available options. If you have not done so already, write at least two posts to your e-mail support list, so that your account is taken off moderation and your post will appear immediately if and when real need arises. Contact with others who have been through Intro will be one of your most essential resources during Intro and die-off. Lay it all out and let your new friends support you through this potentially challenging process!

Items Needed

- All of the items previously mentioned in the *Program Tools: Essential Items* section.
- Fat from the inside of any animal.
- Bones and joints, with or without meat on them.
- Meat (including fish), attached to bones or boneless, preferably free of antibiotics, hormones, etc.
- Enough soup to have upon waking the first morning.
- A constipation remedy—preferably an enema kit, but a magnesium supplement or vitamin C powder are also good options (see the section *Detoxification: Bowel Movements—Constipation*).
- Ingredients for the replenishing drink of your choice (see *Recipes: More Essentials*).
- Eggs, preferably organic and from pastured animals.
- Fish, commercially frozen for two weeks at any point before your preparation date, for your *Fermented Fish* recipe.
- A source of probiotics, such as juice from fermented vegetables (see *Recipes: Ferments*) or rejuvelac.
- Three or more die-off relief bath additives (Epsom salts, apple cider vinegar, and baking soda are the most accessible and affordable for most people).
- Activated charcoal (powder, liquid, or capsules).
- Filtered or mineral water.

- A quality salt, such as sea salt (not table salt).
- Peppercorns (and grinder, if you don't want to simply smash them with a wooden spoon).
- Fresh, whole garlic.
- Fresh, whole ginger root.
- Fresh mint leaves, for tea (optional).
- Fresh chamomile, for tea (optional).
- Honey (optional).
- Soup vegetables, as detailed in the next section. Feel free to chop some before starting; keep each veggie in its own bag, so that each can be introduced separately, and any can be eliminated if intolerance is suspected.

Vegetables in Early Intro

In early Intro, everyone is different when it comes to vegetables. Some can tolerate all cooked, GAPS-friendly vegetables right from the start, while other bodies are much more fussy. I would love to be able to make your life easier by providing a concrete list of what veggies to start with, but it is truly different for everyone. For one person, anything cruciferous triggers gas; for another, these are no problem but carrots pass through undigested. Much of GAPS is trial and error. Yes, this can be very frustrating, but it serves us well in the long run because it teaches us how to really listen to our own bodies. The following are some general thoughts.

The GAPS Intro progression suggests starting with non-fibrous veggies or parts of veggies, so that the digestive tract is not irritated. Cabbage, celery, and the stalks of broccoli, for example, are more fibrous. Some people's systems struggle with onions and leafy greens, even when cooked very well.

If you wish to be very careful, which may be critical for folks with severe intestinal damage (e.g., Crohn's disease), start with just broth, fat, and meat for the first few days, then add one vegetable at a time, introducing each new one not more often than every few days. Carrots and zucchini (peeled and de-seeded) are gentle enough for most people. My body was fine with most vegetables and I thrived on the carbohydrates that a full range of veggies could offer, but the slower approach might be a better fit for some.

For my son and me, I determined our initial vegetable list by looking in our local organic aisles for vegetables I was reasonably familiar with and which I intuited would be both very gentle on our systems and easy to incorporate into a soup without overwhelming it. Thus, we started with broccoli florets and cauliflower florets (not the tough stems or stalks), carrots, peeled ginger root (which may be too fibrous for some), mushrooms, yellow onions, bell peppers, winter squashes, and zucchini. (Interestingly, although broccoli and cauliflower had always given me gas in the past, this did not happen on GAPS' Intro. Perhaps this was because I was not using the fibrous stalks, or perhaps the broth helped the digestion.) I avoided garlic because I wanted to pace our die-off, which I tend to find overwhelming otherwise. I did not have access to green (string) beans. I avoided chard, eggplant, and kale only because I could not fathom how I might use them (I soon learned to incorporate kale and/or chard into almost every stew and spaghetti sauce).

After several weeks we tried, without problem, the following: asparagus, beets, garlic, parsley, string beans, and tomatoes. Approximately six weeks from our start date, we tried raw lettuce, raw cucumber, and juiced carrots. I was fine with these; my son was not. Thus, we removed them and tried them again later. After several more weeks we tested chard, eggplant, and kale without problem.

Of the foods we tried, those which proved problematic for either or both of us early on were cabbage and celery (even when very well-cooked), juiced veggies, and raw veggies. For me, all of these became fine after some more weeks or months of healing. For my son, fermented cabbage became acceptable, but he needed several more months to be able to tolerate non-fermented cabbage and celery. I have continued to be unable to tolerate celeriac, initially tested several months into healing. Even after two years on GAPS, it consistently triggered intense nausea and heat in me. Spinach is problematic for quite a few children, possibly because of its high oxalate content.

I regret that it is not possible to provide a "safe" list of vegetables. Rather, I hope I have given a sense of how different people react to different foods, shared sufficiently the caution with which I proceeded initially, and demonstrated that trial, error, and time do indeed allow for excellent healing and the inclusion of more and more GAPS foods. In the meantime, if you are experiencing a specific health condition, be sure to review the information offered in this Guide's *Health Issues* section. Included there under the different disorders and symptoms are additional notes regarding the use of vegetables and other foods in early healing.

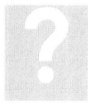

READY?

If you have not yet completed preparing for Intro, as presented in the *Months 1–3: Preparing for Full GAPS/Intro* section of this book, please do so. (If you are choosing not to do the preparation stage despite my strong recommendation, please do at least read through that entire section. There are tips within it relevant to your Intro journey.)

How to Move Through Intro

Be Fully Prepared

Before starting, be sure to read or review all sections of this entire Guide, including those on intolerances and die-off relief. To ease your journey, it will be critical to be familiar with all the contents of this Guide. Whether presented under the *Intro* section or elsewhere, each set of tips will be relevant to Intro, and you will likely need to refer to them regularly.

Eat Only Intro Foods

During Intro, only foods listed within the Intro progression are allowed. Do not eat any other foods. Many people miss the importance of this and include other foods, such as coconut oil (which can pack a real wallop). This can slow healing or trigger great discomfort. Unless you have a compelling reason to do so (and some people may), please avoid the error of including any item not listed in the Intro progression as presented.

Have Frequent Meals

Offer yourself protein and fat—even if just a small amount—upon waking and then every 60 to 90 minutes throughout the day, just before bedtime, and every time you notice you feel hungry. Consider setting an alarm to remind you, so that you don't suddenly find yourself having gone too long without a serving. At each offering, you (or those you are caring for, including children) decide whether and how much to eat. It is not necessary to eat at every offering, but it is important that food is accessible at least this often. This will ensure the rapidly healing body is being sufficiently nourished. It will also keep blood sugar stable. If a person is not eating, ensure they are at least taking an electrolyte drink (not simply water), plus any other replenishing drink they wish throughout the day. Eat as much as your body wants. (Parents may be shocked by the sheer volume of food their children will eat at some points on GAPS. Support their nutritional needs by allowing as much savoury food as the child requests.)

Pacing

The pace at which one moves through Intro will be very individual. For example, you may spend just two days or a full week or (rarely) a month at any point in Intro's Stages 2–6. Also, depending on your sensitivities, you may have to introduce some foods much later (or earlier in rare cases) than outlined.

Determining when to move forward is more an art than a science. For my son, food reactions typically involved any of the following: night wakings, incontinence, extreme and sudden tantrums during which his eyes indicated overwhelm and fear, snaking backward on his belly across the floor, and more. My own standard was to see four days clear of these reactions before introducing a new food. That way, I was not overwhelming his system and I could get a clear indication of which foods might be problematic. As with many people, his stool changes were not a particularly reliable sign, so I learned to ignore these for the most part.

Proceed cautiously with a new food item, amount, style of preparation, or supplement every four days. The only case in which you will pause for longer than that is if you experience an obvious, noticeable reaction to a food, in which case you will remove that food, wait a few days and then move forward to the subsequent item in the progression. For example, if the first point in Intro in which you notice a food reaction is upon introducing soft-boiled eggs in soup, stop adding soft-boiled eggs, return to your tolerated foods (soups and yolks in soups) for another four days, and then move forward to the stews. This approach works very well for many people, allowing them to establish a wider menu—plus renewed vigour and psychological endurance—earlier than they otherwise might. However, you may also choose to remove the problematic food, spend an additional one to two weeks at the last point at which all listed foods were tolerated, then retest the one that had triggered a reaction. The additional digestive rest and healing may or may not have resolved the intolerance. If it hasn't, I suggest moving forward regardless.

REMEMBER

Do not wait for perfection. Not all of your issues will resolve immediately; therefore, except in cases of extreme reactions to Intro foods (e.g., seizures), in which case it will be important to work with a health practitioner familiar with GAPS, you will be moving forward while some issues are still present. Intro can be a confusing process. Simply keep moving forward while communicating regularly with your GAPS supports. Don't worry: As you proceed, you will discover personal signals and guidelines that are effective for you.

Anticipate Intense Die-Off

Expect to experience any one or more of the issues listed under *What to Expect in Intro* and be prepared with a plan, remedy supplies, and support. Also, because it frightens the parents so much, it bears emphasizing that in the first one to five days, quite a few children will experience pallor, extreme lethargy, total loss of appetite, and/or vomiting. Allow your child to rest or play (depending on his preference), ensure he is staying hydrated (see *Recipes: More Essentials–Replenishing Drinks*), and do lots of die-off relief support as detailed under *Relief from Transitional Discomfort*—especially the bowel movements (supported by an enema, if needed) and die-off relief baths. Again, have your GAPS supports in place before the transition, so that you have people to e-mail or phone when you need immediate emotional and psychological support.

Supplements/Bottled Foods

Dr. Campbell-McBride notes that people who started fermented foods, commercial probiotics, or cod liver oil before GAPS or before Intro may continue taking these throughout. It is helpful to be aware that many people find their sensitivity to these increases with Intro. If this may be the case for you (and you generally won't know until after the fact), remove all ferments and bottled food from your diet before starting Intro. Each bottled food (e.g., cod liver oil or probiotic) is introduced in exactly the same way as any unbottled food. That is, each will be introduced four or more days after the introduction of any other food or product, with any reactions observed. Again, people with involuntary movements such as tics or seizures should avoid fish oils and fish liver oils.

I recommend keeping bottled foods out of your program for the first while. This is so that you can focus your "new introductions" on yummier, more versatile foods. A variety of textures and flavours can be critical to our staying with the program. When your diet feels sufficiently varied and interesting, which for most people is not earlier than Stage 3, bottled foods can be introduced at any time from that point onward.

Recipes

For most dishes mentioned in the Intro progression, there is at least one recipe in the *Recipes* section of this Guide. There are copious other sources of GAPS recipes both online and in books, and some include recipes specifically for Intro. Please see this Guide's section *Recipes: More Essentials—More Recipes for Intro and Beyond*. Within the resources provided there, look for options available to you in each stage.

Every Morning

Start the day with:

- A cup of still mineral or filtered water, warm or at room temperature, with 15 mL (1 tablespoon) of apple cider vinegar or a slice of lemon in it. Drink the water slowly, sloshing it around your mouth with a "chewing" motion to draw the healing properties of your saliva into it before swallowing.
- Your probiotic source (once introduced).

You can eat your first meal immediately, if hungry, or as late as 10 AM.

CHAPTER 7

STAGES OF INTRO

Some foods are easier than others for a damaged gut to digest. For most GAPS people, the body can most easily accept foods in the order presented below. In the following sections, I also offer information regarding "time on this stage," "when to move forward," and so on. Although introduced within the Stage 1 segment, this information is largely the same from stage to stage; please refer back to it as you proceed through the subsequent stages.

Stage 1

Time on this Stage

For most people, this stage will last one to three days. However, when cramping, bleeding, or true (potentially dehydrating) diarrhea is present, you will stay on this stage for up to seven days, at which point you will move forward regardless of symptoms. See also *When to Move Forward* at the end of this section.

Foods on this Stage

Please also see the detailed food notes following the bulleted list:

- Short-simmered meat/fish broths.
- Fats, marrow, and soft tissue from the insides of animals.
- Boiled meats (including fish), preferably free of hormones, antibiotics, etc.
- Vegetables, as detailed previously.
- Water, either plain, mineral, electrolyte, or with apple cider vinegar or lemon added. A small amount of carbonated water (perhaps to add fizz to a child's replenishing drink) may be fine if it does not aggravate heartburn or other symptoms. Do not drink unfiltered, chlorinated tap water.
- Honey.
- Sea salt.
- Black peppercorns.
- Garlic, whole fresh.
- Tea made from fresh, whole ginger; fresh mint leaves; or fresh chamomile.

It is a common misunderstanding that Stage 1 of GAPS' Intro includes only broths. This is not correct. As noted previously, you should be taking in at least meats and fats from Day 1 as well as broths. For most people, vegetables can also be enjoyed from the very first day. The Stage 1 foods can be mixed together into soups (if you have completed the steps under *Preparing for Full GAPS/Intro*, you are now very comfortable making these). Alternatively, the various Stage 1 foods can be simmered together or separately—all the items preferably in broth—then served on separate dishes. The meats can be topped with reduced broth, or the vegetables can be puréed for the boiled meat pieces to be dipped into. Meats can be simmered in any form, including ground, chunks, steaks, patties, and so on. Boiled meat balls, perhaps with minced or puréed vegetables mixed within them, are a lovely option. Simmering an abundance of any one vegetable (e.g., cauliflower florets, onions, or butternut squash) in a moderate amount of broth and then blending it with some salt and pepper will make a lovely creamed soup. In this Guide's *Recipes: Soups for Intro* section are sample soup recipes. To locate more Stage 1 recipes, please see this Guide's section *Recipes: More Essentials–More Recipes for Intro and Beyond.*

Broths: Intro's meat broths are simmered for a short period (unlike a bone broth which triggers a reaction in some). If you are reactive to the first broth you try, test one made from a different meat (e.g., salmon, cod, chicken, buffalo, or lamb). Salted, the broth can be taken as a hot or cold drink throughout the day, incorporated into your soups, or reduced to a sauce or dip for meat strips. If your body is already accustomed to bone broth and you are certain you do not react to it, you can continue using bone broths. If you do not tolerate apple cider vinegar, simply omit it from any broth recipe; it is not necessary for a meat broth. For more information, see *Recipes: More Essentials.*

Fats, Marrow, and Tissue: At this stage, and until otherwise noted, fats do not include vegetable oils, ghee, butter, or coconut oil. Fat from the inside of an animal can be rendered at home (see the *Recipes* section) or ordered directly from a natural food store, a butcher, a farmer, or via the Internet. Most people should use a lot of fat. It adds vital nutrition, aids healing, and helps one feel satiated. During periods of intensive healing, I take at least 250 mL (1 cup) each day through fatty soups and by adding additional fat to all food. Some people, such as those who have had their gall bladder removed, may have difficulty tolerating fat initially. In this case, start with a small amount (even 5 mL or 1 teaspoon) and increase the amount as you are able. Also be sure to read the tips under this Guide's section *Health Issues: Fat Malabsorption.* The marrow and soft tissues from around the animals' joints are essential to consume—the more, the better.

Meats: In this early stage, meats (including fish) are not to be fried or baked. Meats are to be boiled or simmered only. Meats are an excellent source of protein, and can be eaten by most people without restriction, but the dietary focus should be on the marrow, soft tissue, gelatin, and fats of the animal, drawn from within the bones and around the meat and joints.

Vegetables: If you do not have cramping, bleeding, true (dehydrating) diarrhea, or a known intolerance to a specific vegetable, any GAPS vegetable can be included. As long as a given vegetable does not trigger other issues (e.g., bloating), it can be included to add variety, flavour, carbohydrates, and nutrients to this early stage of your program. Having given up processed foods, you will notice that carrots, onions, and butternut squash are quite sweet. The sugars in these may trigger blood sugar spikes—with dramatic symptoms—in some people. Start with smaller amounts of these vegetables (preferably in relatively low proportion to broth, fats, meats and less sweet vegetables) and gauge your reactions. At this stage, use the florets of cauliflower and broccoli, but not the tough stems and stalks. As noted in the section of this Guide *Health Issues: Severe Intestinal Issues*, a person with cramping, bleeding, diarrhea, or intolerances to certain vegetables may begin their program with no vegetables or with just easier-to-digest ones, such as zucchini or carrots, and then add a new one every few days. A person with a stronger system, on the other hand, might add a variety of vegetables to the pot right from the start, backtracking only if problems arise. Finally, since most vegetable ferments have high-fibre cabbage as their base, we start with just the juice of these. As tolerances permit, early Intro vegetables may include, among others: broccoli florets, carrots, cauliflower florets, kale, mushrooms, onions, bell peppers, squash (summer and winter), zucchini, and others–in other words, any cooked vegetable on the list of recommended foods that is well tolerated by you.

Water: Water should be taken at room temperature or warm (not cold, as this can aggravate a damaged gut). Although plain or salted water is sufficient for some, many do much better with an enhanced water. Mineral water can prevent and relieve leg cramps. A homemade electrolyte drink sipped over the course of the day can keep a person hydrated, counter the effects of diarrhea, promote bowel movements, reduce die-off intensity, prevent vomiting, and boost one's overall well-being. Detailed information on *Replenishing Drinks* is included in this Guide's *Recipes: More Essentials* section.

Honey: Honey should be severely restricted. I prefer to see it used only as an ingredient in a balanced electrolyte drink. If you can't tolerate this stage of the program without it, 5 mL (1 teaspoon) in a cup of tea or taken directly off a spoon (especially as a reward for a child taking broth or soup) is fine. Aim for as little as possible. I suggest a maximum of 15 mL (1 tablespoon) per day for an adult or struggling child. Rely on carrots and orange squash for any additional sweetness, but if an additional teaspoon or two of honey feels critical, feel free.

Tea: For ginger tea, see the *Recipes: More Essentials* section.

Probiotics: On the one hand, probiotic foods (e.g., fermented vegetables) are essential to introduce from early on. On the other hand, many people find the initial wave of discomfort from dietary changes alone to be very intense. Thus, I suggest that most people start Intro without probiotics added, allow the initial wave of die-off to pass, and only then introduce probiotics. Within the Stage 2 section, I have included a reminder to start these.

Eating

It is important to eat as often as the body requests it, especially in early Intro. For many people, this will be upon waking, every 60 to 90 minutes throughout the day, and again right before bed. Meals may be large or small, but they should be as frequent as the body desires. Stage 1 foods can be eaten together as a soup. Alternatively, the meats, fats, and (if applicable) vegetables can be separated from their cooking broth and eaten as solids along with a cup of broth. While the early stages of GAPS include a limited number of foods, there are ways to achieve at least some degree of variety, so long as you know or expect each of the foods to be tolerated. You might have carrots, chicken (with its marrow, fat, and soft tissues), and broth in separate bowls for your breakfast meal; cauliflower florets, beef (with its marrow, fat, and soft tissues), and broth mixed together in one bowl for your mid-morning snack; mushrooms and salmon for your lunch meal; and so on. Personally, I find it easiest to make one giant soup in the morning and eat some of that for breakfast, fill insulated food containers with it for lunch and snacks, and refrigerate the rest for supper.

Children may refuse food for one to five days. This is fine, but they must be kept hydrated, which requires not just water, but electrolytes (see *Recipes: More Essentials–Replenishing Drinks*). An adult, too, may experience a world of difference by including one or more replenishing drinks in their Intro. These can maintain balances of potassium, magnesium, and so on, which can prove vital to one's sense of well-being, eliminate extraneous symptoms, and prevent serious issues such as dehydration. If possible, use a replenishing drink that is stage-friendly, but if there is not a stage-friendly one that meets your immediate need, use any of the options listed in that section.

When to Move Forward

If you started Intro free of cramping, bleeding, or true (dehydrating) diarrhea, move forward after one to three days, based on your personal preference. That is, if you are loving Stage 1, feel free to stay on it for a maximum of 3 days, but if you are eager to move forward after just 1 day, do so.

On the other hand, if you started Intro with cramping, bleeding, or true diarrhea, move forward whenever these resolve or after seven days, whichever comes first. That is, if cramping, bleeding, or true diarrhea persists into Day 7, move forward at that point regardless (be sure to review the tips listed under this Guide's section *Health Issues: Severe Intestinal Issues*).

Regardless of which symptoms you had when you began Intro, during and after Stage 1 you will very likely have at least some of the symptoms you started with, if not all of them. While some people will indeed experience relief of some symptoms within the first few days, the full healing in GAPS does not occur simply upon removing some foods; the healing occurs through a paced, methodical progression of healing the gut—which takes time—and the progressive addition of nutrient-dense, healing foods. While some symptoms may disappear almost immediately; others may take weeks, months, or even the entire two-year program to resolve. Some people are tempted to stay on Stage 1 indefinitely, believing more healing will be achieved, but there is no need to stay on this stage longer than specified, and it is vital to your physical health and psychological interest to move forward.

REMEMBER

Stage 1, and Intro in general, will not make us symptom-free. Continue moving forward despite the persistence of some symptoms.

Stage 2

From this stage forward, you will continue applying the guidelines provided for Stage 1. You will simply add a new food, in the order presented, about every four days. If you know that you have an intolerance to a food listed in the Intro progression, or you are uncomfortable introducing a specific food for any reason, simply skip it and move to the next item. However, as each food listed is highly nutritious and healing, minimize omissions as much as possible, preferably doing so only when a food is specifically not tolerated by your body.

Introduce each item cautiously and progressively. For example, cooked apple purée should be started with a few spoonfuls on its first day and slowly increased from there if there is no reaction.

Time on this Stage

Most people will spend one to three weeks on this (and each subsequent) stage of Intro. A relatively small number of people experience their best health on this stage and for a time experience a return of severe problems (e.g., seizures) with anything beyond it. If you are one of these rare people, you will stay on this stage longer (in this case, it is also especially advisable to work with a health practitioner familiar with GAPS).

Foods on this Stage

Continue all Stage 1 foods and guidelines while adding one new item at a time in the following order. Add a new food, style of preparation, or supplement about every four days. If you experience an obvious reaction to a new introduction, stop the newly introduced item, return to your immediately previous range of foods until symptoms subside, then move to the subsequent item in the list.

- **Raw egg yolk** from pastured animals or from truly free-range animals fed all-organic feed, added to soup or meat stock. Many people are put off by the idea of yolk in their soup, but whisked in it gives the soup a softer, creamier consistency that many people discover they enjoy very much. Start with one egg yolk per day. While also moving forward with the rest of Intro, gradually increase the amount until you are having an egg yolk with every bowl of soup. If you are concerned about raw eggs and salmonella, please see Dr. Campbell-McBride's presentation about this in her book *Gut and Psychology Syndrome* or check in with one of the support lists.

If you experience a negative change in your body in response to a non-probiotic food (e.g., diarrhea or a return of any previous symptom), stop eating just that food, and continue to enjoy all the foods previously introduced. When symptoms subside, or after four days, move on to the subsequent food in the progression. Retest the troublesome food after two or more weeks; otherwise continue with the progression, moving ever forward.

- **Soft-boiled (whites cooked and yolks still runny) eggs** in the soups. People often ask at this point in the progression if they can skip ahead to hard-boiled. Please remember that every item in the progression is there for a reason. Unless your individual situation dictates otherwise, the foods should be progressed through as presented; each supports progressive healing while not overwhelming the body. As with all Intro foods, once tolerance is established, eggs may be unlimited in quantity.

Shortly after this point, usually around Day 5 or so of your program, you may find that the initial wave of discomfort (if any) has passed. The timing of this shift is different for everyone, but once it occurs, introduce your initial dose of probiotic, usually 5 mL (1 teaspoon) or less of juice from your home-fermented vegetables. (If no juice is visible, simply press your spoon horizontally into the batch until some flows into the spoon.) If you previously eliminated dairy for 2-6 weeks and subsequently reintroduced it without problem, and you choose to include dairy in your Intro, feel free to use homemade whey as your first probiotic source, starting with 5 mL (1 teaspoon) or less (whey may be especially helpful in cases of diarrhea). Make sure your food is not too hot (i.e., no hotter than the original fermentation temperature) when adding probiotic foods to it because excess heat will destroy the beneficial bacteria. A simple system for increasing your probiotic is to increase (perhaps doubling) the dose on a specific day each week (e.g., every Saturday). Follow this pattern until you can add a few teaspoons of the probiotic food into every cup of meat stock and bowl of soup. If you cannot tolerate the juice from fermented vegetables, feel free to introduce a commercial probiotic. For more information about the use of probiotics, be sure to read the *Supplementation: Probiotics* section of this Guide. As noted there, for your comfort it is essential to introduce probiotic foods or powder very gradually. People who are very sensitive, very ill, or very young may need to start with even less than suggested—such as the amount of yogurt that lies on the tip of a dipped butter knife, or just a spoonful of water from a cup containing one-tenth of a capsule of commercial probiotic. Slow and steady wins the race!

In preparation for your fermented fish, thaw the fish.

- **Stews** (simply a thicker, heartier, longer-simmered, meat-inclusive soup) and **casseroles** made with meats, vegetables, salt, and **fresh (only) herbs**, with some probiotic food added to each serving. For maximum healing, include as much fat as possible with these.

Two days before you plan to proceed to the next step, begin preparing your fermented fish. Many people are tempted to skip this step, as I did my first time. After I finally tried it, I found it simple to make and lovely to eat. Although it may seem intimidating, I strongly recommend including this step in your Intro progression.

- **Fermented fish or Swedish gravlax**, starting with one piece a day and gradually increasing. The recipe in this Guide (see *Recipes: Ferments–Fermented Fish*) was adapted from material by Dr. Campbell-McBride and includes whey. Most people reach this stage of Intro not sooner than two weeks into the program, which has so far been dairy-free. Thus, this is generally an appropriate time to test one's tolerance of whey. If you are choosing not to test any form of dairy yet, you can make the Swedish gravlax, as presented in the book *Gut and Psychology Syndrome*.

Remember: After a two-week break from any food listed so far which triggered a reaction for you, feel free to retest it. For tips, see this Guide's section *Food Issues: Food Sensitivities/Allergies*.

- The fermented fish recipe offered by Dr. Campbell-McBride includes **dried herbs and spices** in addition to Stage 1's peppercorns. At this point in Intro, most bodies can accommodate any dried herbs and spices in any dish or tea. As many commercial sources of tea include chicory, soy, etc., it is best to use leaves grown and/or dried locally. Commercial spices may be tolerated, but be sure to look for ones that have no non-GAPS ingredients. Mixed spices sometimes include flowing agents, so single spices are preferred (and may prove critical for those with severe digestive issues).

REMEMBER

At any point in the Intro progression, you might find your body experiences wonderful health, but struggles with anything presented subsequently. If this is true for you, don't worry. As long as you are having fats, soft tissues, marrow, gelatin, protein (eggs, meat, or fish), probiotics, and (ultimately) juiced vegetables, this combination will sustain you nutritionally and allow for healing to occur. A wider range of foods will be successfully reintroduced over time, providing for greater variety and the psychological enjoyment that comes with that.

- **Homemade ghee**, starting with 5 mL (1 teaspoon) a day and gradually increasing. Note that even if you do not yet tolerate whey or other dairy, you may still tolerate ghee because it is free of most of dairy's aggravating elements. Ghee will add gorgeous flavour to all your dishes. Add it to stews, salmon, soups, and so on. As you progress through the stages, you can also spread it onto any firm food.

A note about supplements: I like to see people reach at least this point before starting even one of the bottled foods. This is because if we devote four to seven days to the introduction of each bottled food—rather than to another non-bottled food (e.g., eggs or ghee)—we can find ourselves stuck with a very limited variety of meal options. I suggest you work up to a stage of Intro that feels sufficiently varied and interesting for you and introduce bottled foods at that point, if not later. So, if you feel your diet is now varied enough to prevent boredom, feel free to introduce your first GAPS supplement. Ideally, start with a commercial probiotic (if you did not do so earlier) and, over time, introduce cod liver oil, then fish oil, then olive oil, and then nut/seed oil. Whether introducing a bottled food this early or waiting until you have reached Full GAPS to do so, simply add each one as you would any other food (i.e., at least four days after the introduction of any other food, starting with a very small amount, watching for reactions, stopping it if there's an issue, then moving forward to the next item in the progression). If the bottled food is tolerated, build your dose slowly. Alternatively, the supplements can be introduced after completing Intro and at any point during Full GAPS in this same way.

When to Move Forward

Again, simply add another food, style of preparation, or supplement about every four days. Upon introducing the final item listed under Stage 2 (i.e., ghee), wait about four days then move on to the first item (i.e., avocado) presented under Stage 3.

Stage 3

People are often relieved and joyous to reach this stage, with its creamy, fresh avocado and nut butter!

Foods on this Stage

- **Ripe avocado mashed into soups**, starting with 5–15 mL (1–3 teaspoons) and gradually increasing the amount.

- **Nut butter pancakes/crêpes**, starting with one per day and gradually increasing the amount. Many of us delight in the new flavour and texture offered by the pancakes and overdo our consumption, while others react to even a small amount of the nut butter (quite possibly to its carbohydrate content). Make a small batch of the pancakes and freeze them, eating only one per day initially.

Although not listed within the Intro progression, eggs poached in broth, soft-boiled eggs outside of soups, and eggs lightly fried in lots of fat may be well tolerated at this stage. Meat cakes (previously simmered meat or fish now blended with eggs, formed into patties, and grilled in lots of fat) are also often well tolerated at this stage. Feel free to test each of these, one at a time, with at least four days between each addition.

- **Eggs scrambled** with plenty of ghee, goose fat, or duck fat. Serve with avocado and cooked vegetables. Many people, including my son in his early healing, experience some difficulty with scrambled eggs. If this proves true for you, stick with the previously introduced preparation styles, move forward, and retest scrambled eggs later.

- **Cooked onion**. Melt 75 mL (5 tablespoons) of animal fat in a pan. Add one large, sliced white onion. Cover. Cook for 20–30 minutes on low heat. Enjoy this as a side dish to meat or eggs, or use them as the foundation for a soup. Dr. Campbell-McBride notes that this dish is particularly good for the digestive and immune systems. From this point forward, onions and garlic may be sautéed for 20 minutes for any soup or dish, adding an increased depth of flavour.

> ### REMEMBER
> Once you have progressed from a soup vegetable's 30-minute simmer to the onion's 20-minute sauté, you can slowly begin to reduce cooking times for all vegetables. Over several subsequent weeks, you can test progressively shorter cooking times as preferred for specific dishes.

- **Home-fermented vegetables**. You have been taking the juice from this already; now you will test the fibrous part of the batch. Start with a small amount and gradually increase to 15–60 mL (1–4 tablespoons) per meal. To preserve the probiotic content, serve it on a cooler part of your plate.

When to Move Forward

Upon completing this stage, simply move on approximately four days after having tested the fermented vegetables to the first item presented under the next stage.

Stage 4

Foods on this Stage

- **Meats can now be roasted, baked, or grilled** (but not barbecued or fried yet). A roasted chicken is nice at this stage, and grilled fish brings a welcome change in texture. Avoid parts which are burned or very brown. Eat the meat with cooked vegetables and fermented vegetables, as your personal tolerances allow.

Although not listed within the Intro progression, plain omelettes (i.e., no cheese or veggies) may be tolerated at this stage. Cook in lots of animal fat (among its many benefits, the inclusion of copious animal fats has resolved intolerance of high-sulphur foods in many).

- **Cold-pressed olive oil.** Add to meals, starting with a few drops per meal. Gradually increase the amount to 15–30 mL (1–2 tablespoons) per meal.

- **Freshly pressed juices**, starting with approximately 45 mL (3 tablespoons) of carrot juice diluted in warm water (or whey or yogurt), sipped slowly, swishing and "chewing" each mouthful before swallowing. Drink the juice on an empty stomach (e.g., first thing in the morning). This point in Intro is challenging for many. Start small; move slowly. Make sure that the juice is clear (fibre-free); filter it well. Start with a very small amount and work up. (If you do not already have a juicer, you might access the small amount needed initially by simply blending the vegetables in a strong food processor, then pressing their juices out through a nut milk bag or cheesecloth.) The juices are detoxifying, the effect of which may be felt, but if the juice is carrot-based or fruit-enhanced, the natural sugars—not slowed by fibre—may also trigger a reaction in some people. If this is the case for you, you have at least two options: (1) experiment with vegetables such as celery and cucumber or (2) skip this step for now and after sour cream or coconut oil are successfully introduced in Full GAPS, whisk two raw eggs plus sour cream or coconut oil with the juice to support a reaction-free absorption. Gradually increase juice to 250 mL (1 cup) per day. When a full cup of carrot juice is well tolerated, add to it juice from celery, cabbage, lettuce, and fresh mint leaves. As you become accustomed to juices, review the section of this Guide on *Detoxification: Juicing* for more information, including the ultimate intake goal.

Whether or not you have been able to include every single food listed so far, if you are consuming marrow, soft tissues, and fats from the inside of animals, protein (meats, fish, or eggs), juiced vegetables, and a probiotic food, your diet is now sufficiently well-rounded. Some people—including those sensitive to carbohydrates or those wanting to launch a greater attack on *Candida* overgrowth—choose not to proceed with the steps involving fruit, flour-centred baking, or increased honey until a later time.

Baked goods made from flour (even almond or coconut) are problematic for a number of people: the high-fibre content of these may trigger issues such as bloating or diarrhea—eating fermented foods such as kefir alongside baked goods may make all the difference. Even when baked goods are not particularly problematic in and of themselves, the familiar and comforting texture of these foods may lead one to begin to rely too heavily on them, reducing the amount and variety of other nutrient-dense foods in one's diet.

If any of these issues apply to you, feel free to exclude the fruit, flour-centred baking, or increased honey for a time. Alternatively, build up to a wide range of GAPS foods, and then exclude any you feel may be hindering your healing. If doing either approach, please do not exclude too many foods unnecessarily. You will need to eat something after all! Also, variety can be key to remaining on the program. Even people initially sensitive to carbohydrates may need to add some back in for energy and weight balancing once that issue is healed.

If you are comfortable proceeding exactly as presented, do so. The raw, crispy, whole vegetables are especially appreciated at this point; most find these very refreshing. These and all the other remaining foods add variety, flavour, and additional nutrition, and are indeed well tolerated by many at this point.

- **GAPS bread.** Start with a small piece and gradually increase the amount. As with the nut butter pancakes, most of us overdo this one. Bake a very small batch, cut off one slice per person, and freeze the rest. For many people, the nuts or seeds used in the breads must be properly soaked (see *Recipes: More Essentials–Nuts and Seeds*). Commercial nut flours are handy and versatile, making life on GAPS much easier, but for many people nut flours are the most difficult nut products to digest, often leaving the sensation of a rock in one's tummy. I do not know of any commercial nut flour that is soaked before processing. For a number of people, commercial nut flours must be delayed for several months. Home-soaked or fermented nuts and seeds and commercial nut butters are often tolerated in the interim.

Stage 5

Foods on this Stage

Although not listed in Intro, the short-cooked vegetables in an omelette (cooked in lots of animal fat) may be tolerated now. At this point, you may also be able to tolerate more sources and amounts of fibre (e.g., leafy greens and broccoli stalks) in each soup, stew, or casserole.

- **Cooked apple purée.** Peel and core ripe cooking apples and stew them with a bit of water until soft. When they are cooked, add a generous amount of ghee, duck fat, or goose fat and mash it all with a potato masher. Start with a few spoonfuls each day. Watch for any reaction. If there is none, gradually increase the amount.

- Raw vegetables, starting with a small amount of **soft lettuce parts and peeled cucumber**. The fibre content may trigger bloating or stool changes. Allow time for your body to adjust, maintaining the "low and slow" approach to introducing foods. When those two vegetables are well tolerated, gradually add **other raw vegetables**: carrot, tomato, cabbage, and so on. Be sure to chew them well.

- If juice made from carrot, celery, lettuce, and mint is well tolerated, start **adding fruit to the juice** (e.g., apple, pineapple, and mango). Avoid citrus fruit at this stage.

Stage 6

Foods on this Stage

- If all the foods introduced so far are well tolerated, add **peeled raw apple** (chew it well).
- Add **any other raw fruit**.
- Increase the amount of **honey**, if desired.
- Add **cakes and other permitted sweets**, if desired.

Moving to Full GAPS

Any food not listed in Intro is not to be used during Intro. It can, however, be tested any time after Intro is completed. Once the above stages are completed and your main symptoms have subsided, move methodically into Full GAPS, ultimately including all relevant supplements, too. At any point, introduce any Full GAPS food you wish, preferably using the same method you used to introduce each of the Intro foods (i.e., starting with a small amount, watching for a reaction, and building up slowly).

Ensure you are taking at least 250 mL (1 cup) of soup or broth daily for the duration of your healing (and preferably beyond). Work up to 500 mL (2 cups) of freshly pressed juices daily. As you continue to add foods over the course of your program, ensure that every week the vast majority of your foods are savoury ones (e.g., marrow, soft tissues, fats from the inside of animals, meats, fish, eggs, organs, ferments, dairy, and vegetables).

The following foods trigger issues in a number of people and should be approached with awareness. If a food proves problematic for you, simply remove the food from your program and retest it regularly per the information in the *Food Issues: Food Sensitivities/Allergies* section. For those for whom a reaction is due to a food's carbohydrate count, you may be able to successfully implement limited (or unlimited) portions of these foods after some months restricting carbohydrates (for more information, see this Guide's section *Food Issues: Assess Carbohydrate Sensitivity*). Again, except where an actual intolerance is present, the following foods should not be avoided unnecessarily. The nutrition, flavour, and variety they offer are important to the program!

- **Coconut oil:** Coconut oil is a very powerful food, thus an excellent healer. Taking it during Intro often greatly exacerbates a person's transitional discomfort. Although not listed in Intro, many people take it at that time anyway. I strongly recommend delaying the introduction of coconut oil until after Intro has been completed and you are free of discomfort. When you do introduce it, start with 5 mL (1 teaspoon) or less per day and build up slowly.

- **Dairy:** A guide to the consideration, elimination, and reintroduction of dairy is offered in the *Food Issues: Dairy* section.

- **Beans (white, navy, haricot, and lima), lentils, and split peas:** Several months into the program, you may be able to incorporate GAPS beans, lentils, and split peas. These can help reduce your food budget and add variety in taste and texture. Ferment them according to *Recipes: Ferments– Beans, Proper Preparation* section.

- **Higher-fibre veggies:** Turnips, broccoli stalks, celery, etc., can aggravate a damaged gut. Intro may have provided enough healing for these to be included now. You may test them any time after Intro is completed, but feel free to delay them another few months, too.

- **Foods that do not appear in the list of recommended foods:** There are exceptions. See this Guide's section *Diet: What to Eat and When—Additional Foods.*

CHAPTER 8

ADDRESSING CHALLENGES

Resolving Common Mistakes

Here is a list of the most common errors. Review this list at the time of any challenge. It can potentially save you from unnecessary frustration, suffering, and/or expense.

Skipping bowel movements: When people describe any suffering, one of my first questions is: "How often are you ensuring a bowel movement?" Bowel movements should occur one to three times daily. When this does not happen, toxins are held—and continue to circulate—within your body. It is critical to release these. When an enema is required, it will be well worth it, but there are many other movement encouragers that can be implemented, too. Review the tips under *Detoxification: Bowel Movements—Constipation* section and try each one in turn—starting with whichever you prefer that falls within your current stage—each for four days in a row. After diet, ensuring one to three bowel movements daily may be the most critically important aspect to the program. Nevertheless, I receive posts from so many people who say they are simply not following this tip. I cannot emphasize enough the importance of this point: If we are not releasing the contents of our bowels daily, toxins are churning in our systems and being reintegrated into our bodies. This will not only prevent healing, it will make us feel awful in the meantime. For healing to occur, daily bowel movements must take place. Granted, even while doing one's utmost to ensure bowel movements, there will be days when none will occur. That's okay! But this should happen rarely, not be the norm.

Probiotics: Problems can occur if you start probiotics at too high a dose (even half a capsule), or increase the dose too quickly. Many people coming to GAPS miss or disregard this note and suffer needlessly as a result. Please carefully review the information on probiotics in the *Supplementation: Probiotics* section.

Skipping the detoxifying/die-off relief baths: The baths can be critical to healing and for maintaining a feeling of wellness during the healing process. See *Detoxification: Die-Off Relief Baths*.

Skipping Intro indefinitely: I do recommend delaying Intro until after you have spent at least 1 month transitioning to the program and then an additional several weeks enjoying Full GAPS. However, Intro is still important to do! The gains can be tremendous. After completing the *Preparing for Full GAPS/Intro* steps, do choose a date within the next six months or so to start Intro.

Avoiding foods indefinitely: As noted within the *Food Issues: Food Sensitivities/Allergies* section, we must not underestimate the body's capacity to heal. A food you could not tolerate in Week 1, 7, or 12 may become well-accepted by the body after a few more weeks or months of healing. That food may be critical to achieving one's next level of health. Widening one's physical capacity for nourishing foods is one of the main purposes of GAPS. Be sure to retest foods and incorporate as many of GAPS' nutrient-dense foods as possible over time.

Relying on sweets, treats, and common fare: When we come to GAPS, we often attempt to create a GAPS version of our previous diet. Thus, we make breads, cakes, and cookies, skip breakfast because we don't know what GAPS foods fit for this meal, and so on. This approach feeds cravings for sugar and limits healing. Over the course of a week, a good 85% of most GAPSters' diets (enjoyed as three to six meals daily) should be marrow, soft tissues, fats from the inside of animals, meats, fish, eggs, organs, GAPS dairy, ferments, and vegetables. For most people, fruits, nuts, and seeds should be very limited (though not entirely).

Replenishing drink: As simple as it sounds, this may prove critical to moving toxins out, supporting the body through ketosis or die-off, and ensuring you get needed fluids or salts. See *Recipes: More Essentials–Replenishing Drinks*.

Pushing oneself: Some folks come to this intensive healing program while attempting to maintain their previously established lifestyle of exercise, excess work, and so on. Healing demands a lot of energy. It is critically important to support your body with physical and mental rest. If you have vacation days due, use them in early Intro. If it is possible for your kids to homeschool while they are doing Intro, consider this option. If you can release some expenses (e.g., cable TV, a vehicle, a fitness pass, or new clothing) in order to reduce your hours at work, do so. If a relationship is causing tension, access mediation or counselling or consider ending it. Do not underestimate the impact of physical, emotional, and logistical stress on your capacity to heal! The good news is that in addressing these lifestyle challenges, your healing will prove synergistic, bringing astounding healing at many levels. See the tips under *Limited Energy* and *Limited Time*.

Maintaining old habits: Again, we sometimes approach GAPS as merely a different grocery list, but try to keep our lives otherwise the same. For example, we might attempt to continue our pre-GAPS approaches of eating only three times per day, restricting our fat intake, exercising vigorously, drinking 2 litres of water per day, filling every school lunch bag with a sandwich and juice, and so on.

In most cases, this approach doesn't work. After some healing, you might find one or more of these former habits (such as vigorous movement) to be appropriate to your personal program, but each will need to be re-assessed for you as an individual and in relation to your intention of healing. In other words, we need to recognize how different GAPS is from a conventional approach to health and realize that our relationship with meal frequency, exercise, water intake, sleep, and everything else will shift along with our diet. Many common beliefs, and our previous understandings and practices, will no longer apply.

Combining with other programs: Most people coming to GAPS have done a lot of research. We've read about, and often tried, any or all of: vegetarianism, veganism, food combining, raw food diet, anti-*Candida* diet, low-carb, restricted calorie, fasting, restricted frequency of meals, not eating for two hours before bed, no dairy, and so on. I believe that every body is different, that every program has potential benefits, and that different approaches work best in our bodies at different times and under different circumstances. I also believe that every program is synergistic within itself; that is, that the various aspects of any given program work together to bring maximum benefit. When we implement one aspect from one program, one aspect from another, and a third aspect from yet another, our program can become too cumbersome, burdensome, and restrictive. For example, we may end up attempting a low-fat, dairy-free, three-meals-per-day "GAPS" when our body may actually require a high-fat, dairy-rich, six-meals-per-day program. For both physical and psychological reasons, a mix-and-match may prove both unsustainable and depleting in the long term, rather than healing and nourishing. My suggestion is to choose one program—whether GAPS or a different one—and commit to it 100%, as presented, for at least three to six months before assessing its effectiveness. Positive results will encourage you to continue any given program; poor results can inspire you to select a different program that you can commit 100% to for the subsequent three to six months. In other words, if you choose a raw vegan diet, do that 100%, but if you choose GAPS, do it as presented, eliminating any additional restrictions not dictated to you by your body. (Note that GAPS as presented is already anti-*Candida* and also incorporates raw foods, juicing, and every required nutrient.)

Mimicking another's program: Early in GAPS, it makes sense to follow others' leads. After 3 months or so on GAPS, our own intuition and body signals will become more reliable. At that point, it is important to begin letting go of others' ways and developing your own personal protocol. If one GAPS blogger is eating massive amounts of raw greens every day, but your body craves meat soups, go with your body. The GAPS community consists of people of all ages, heritages, financial means, cultures, religions, and health histories living in various environments and climates. What one person needs is not necessarily what you need.

Ignoring the body's leads: While we are ill, our senses can be off track. After the initial 3 months or so on the program, your body will begin to send you more reliable signals about its needs. One month, it may ask you for more dairy. Another month, it may ask you for more salad. Shortly before each menstrual period, it may ask you for more liver. Rather than rigidly sticking with a pre-determined menu, follow your body's requests. Of course, when caring for another person, such as a young child, it will be more challenging to follow this tip. Under the section *Special Considerations: GAPS Through Life's Stages—Children*, I offer a "buffet" strategy to address this somewhat.

Focusing on input vs. output: Despite our best efforts, our body will feel out of balance at times. We might then diligently add this or that to our diet, aiming to re-establish an optimal sense of well-being. At some points, though, our body may actually be in need of respite. That is, we may need to focus not on what we're eating, but rather on what we're expelling. On these days, skipping meals, sipping lots of water with raw apple cider vinegar added to it, having a detox bath, going for a gentle walk, ensuring one to three bowel movements, and having a good nap or sleep may bring the balance desired. Activated charcoal may also help. In some health circumstances, Dr. Campbell-McBride also recommends brief periods of fasting (for more information, please see Dr. Campbell-McBride's FAQ document).

Relying only on diet: Diet is critically important to health, but other things can also "make or break" our well-being. Emotional stress, a mouldy environment, second-hand cigarette smoke, persistent loneliness, absence of touch, chronic fear, and more will impact us, too. In your effort to heal, focus initially on diet, but once you have found your dietary groove, start to address other aspects of your life. For example, throw out a mouldy carpet, change cubicles at work to be further away from the office's smoking area, get a massage, pursue counselling, end a toxic relationship, join a support group, incorporate occupational therapy for a visual-spatial imbalance, and so on. Be aware that taking on too much at once will create its own stress—try just one thing at a time, starting with a good six months of diet and then give each adjunct therapy at least one month to take effect.

Moving forward too quickly: In our desire to heal more quickly, we may be tempted to implement additional foods, supplements, or protocols too early or with little time between them. Ironically, this can slow healing more than moving slowly in the first place! For example, we may start Intro, then four weeks in feel frustrated by persistent issues, so add an antifungal protocol. In a limited number of cases, and under the care of a health practitioner, this may be the correct route, but for the vast majority of us, stepping gently, slowly, and methodically through healing is the most effective way to go. See *Practical Considerations: Impatience.*

Moving forward too slowly: The foods included in the GAPS list are recommended for good reason. They provide vital nourishment, energy, and satisfaction. Our previous reactions have made many of us fearful to add additional foods. Trust your body's ability to heal through the program; continue to add more foods over time. If you are reactive to a number of foods, implement the tips under *Food Issues: Food Sensitivities/Allergies.*

Coconut oil: Although not listed in the GAPS Intro, many people include it in that phase. This often triggers intense die-off. Keep coconut oil out of your diet and off of your skin until the initial stages of die-off and healing have passed.

Expecting to heal in the first 1–12 months: Again, the program requires a minimum of 18–24 months. Many people do experience relief of most or all symptoms in the first weeks or months, but others do not. Some people experience a much slower, quieter healing and only become aware of their gains after attempting to reintroduce non-GAPS foods and re-experiencing their previous level of debilitation as a result. A few people might not see significant signs of healing for the first 12 months or more! The process can be supported, but not rushed or bypassed.

Believing we're unique: We are all unique in our preferences, needs, expressions, and so on. At the same time, when we view our health circumstance as totally isolated we can run into problems. Every condition and symptom you have experienced has been experienced by someone else on the planet…and very likely by someone else doing GAPS! People often describe their circumstances to me as so unique that they must require adaptations never before needed by anyone else on GAPS. The truth is, most of us coming to GAPS had health experiences that seemed to be bizarre, unusual, uncommon, or rare, but they were actually shared by many others coming to the program. If you truly believe or know your circumstance to be unusual even within the GAPS community, please contact a health practitioner familiar with GAPS. Otherwise, share your experiences and concerns on one of the support lists for mutual encouragement and tip-sharing. You may be amazed at the gains you make upon implementing the program as is while also incorporating the tips gleaned from people who have experienced similar challenges.

Unexplained Relapse

In most cases, a significant recurrence of symptoms, or a "relapse," is due to:

- Eating foods outside of GAPS, or outside of one's current stage;
- Incorporating foods too advanced for one's system;
- Eating a given food in higher quantities than one's body can handle;
- Avoiding proper introductions of foods and supplements; or
- Taking supplements with ingredients not recommended for GAPS patients.

If you are experiencing a relapse and none of the above applies, there is another possible explanation. In *Breaking the Vicious Cycle*, Elaine Gottschall wrote:

> *At about the second or third month, there is sometimes a relapse even when the diet has been carefully followed. This can occur if a person develops a respiratory illness or for no obvious reason. Do not allow this to discourage you! Once the individual gets over this, improvement is usually steady with minor setbacks occurring occasionally during the first year.*

For some people this temporary relapse occurs every two to three months for the first year or so (it is usually less intense each time). There are a number of theories about this issue. One is that these are periods in which the program is taking on the really strong bugs and they, in turn, are fighting for their lives. According to this theory it is especially crucial to adhere to the program during these times. The simplest way to do so is to spend a few days on Stage 1 of Intro (e.g., fatty soups made from gelatinous meat and joints plus well-cooked, tolerated veggies) while also continuing your current dose of probiotics. All of the other tips under *Relief from Transitional Discomfort* will also help very much.

Regarding the potential impact of a virus, Dr. Abram Hoffer noted a similar phenomenon. He cautioned me that despite overall wellness, a cold or flu could bring back "mental" illness in full glory. This issue also declines in intensity as healing progresses. (Conversely, in many children, we find that an active cold or flu virus temporarily suspends many autistic symptoms!)

REMEMBER

A regression is transient. Stick with the program and you will find yourself leaping ahead shortly. The "ugh" is frustrating and can be a real blow to one's will, but it is temporary. Also, the gains experienced immediately following each relapse tend to be significant to dramatic!

When to Consult or Test

In this Guide we address: preparing for healing, doing Intro, detoxifying throughout the program, addressing common mistakes, and determining food sensitivities, among other things. These provide a solid foundation, allowing you to approach the bulk of the program independently. But what if you have followed all these steps and are still experiencing issues? Or what if you feel so overwhelmed and foggy that even selecting your next modification feels beyond you?

Many of us fear treading unfamiliar ground alone. We naturally look to others for information, comfort, troubleshooting, reassurance, and tips. Rightly so, as we are indeed far more successful when we do! Happily, most of these needs are covered through this Guide plus the free online support lists, blogs, comments, GAPS phone pool, and more; indeed, the vast majority of us have done GAPS using only these supports. As mentioned earlier in this Guide, I strongly recommend that every person coming to GAPS sign up with every resource they feel a connection with before problems occur. Doing so can help keep your GAPS journey doable without too much extra expense.

When might one connect with a health practitioner familiar with GAPS? To keep expenses to a minimum (so that you can keep buying food), I suggest a consult when:

- You have a concern about a symptom;
- You have a question about any aspect of the program and it is unanswered within this Guide, within Dr. Campbell-McBride's FAQ document, or within any other GAPS resource, such as those listed within the *Support for You* page on the GAPSguide.com website;
- You have completed several months of GAPS as outlined, including the tips listed under *Progressing Further*, and you still feel stuck;
- You have completed several months of GAPS as outlined, including the tips listed under *Progressing Further*, and you are curious about whether tests might reveal specific imbalances;

- Anxiety about "not knowing it all" is interfering with your ability to do the program;
- No one on any list or blog has experienced, or been able to address, your concern; or
- You feel the need for one knowledgeable and reliably available person to personally walk you through the process.

Remember: If you are experiencing any concerning symptom, be sure to access appropriate medical care. GAPS is not anti-medicine. With the sheer number of people doing GAPS today, odds dictate that some will experience a life-threatening issue at some point, just as a percentage of those within the general population will. In cases of Crohn's disease, schizophrenia, etc., people have successfully aligned excellent medical care (e.g., surgery or medication) with their long-term nutritional approach for wonderful results. We need not choose only one or the other (see *Health Issues: Medication*).

The majority of people coming to GAPS feel confused or overwhelmed initially (that's why this Guide was written), while also experiencing very troubling symptoms (that's why they have come to GAPS). Our emotional, psychological, or physical experience is not unique to us. Most of the time, someone else in the GAPS community has experienced what you are going through and will happily offer reassurance, observations, and tips. Again, be sure to connect with the free support resources before starting, so that they are in place for you if issues arise, and also connect with appropriate medical care as your circumstances dictate.

For an ever-expanding list of health practitioners (e.g., general physicians, naturopaths, osteopaths, and nutritionists) who are familiar with GAPS, please see the *Support for You* page on the GAPSguide.com website. Please note that some health practitioners actively promoting GAPS may suggest variations. One suggestion that causes me much concern is the one to "skip Intro." Despite initially skipping the Intro progression, person after person reports vastly improved results by going back and doing it. Please feel free to access support and guidance from the practitioner of your choice, but please also take Dr. Campbell-McBride's Intro recommendations seriously.

Testing for imbalances: I'm not a fan of testing for imbalances except when symptoms or a health practitioner indicate specific need. For one, testing can be quite expensive and often does not lead to any recommendation beyond the usual GAPS protocol. This is money lost unnecessarily. Secondly, testing tends to be indicative of the body's current picture; that is, it can reflect what was most recently eaten or cleared, which may not accurately represent the person's overall state. Thirdly, testing can lead us on a bit of a wild goose chase, trying to resolve one identified imbalance after another, while the GAPS program is intended to achieve this anyway by bringing the body slowly and gently into balance. The only situations in which I personally would pursue any testing are: (1) if there is concern that the issue may demand urgent or emergency care, or (2) after three to six months of implementing the full healing protocol—including Intro—significant issues remain and it is believed more information may allow those to be addressed. If testing is of interest to you, consider approaching it in cooperation with a health care practitioner, preferably one familiar with GAPS. She will provide test recommendations as well as help you to interpret and respond to the results.

CHAPTER 9
PROGRESSING FURTHER

Have you been doing GAPS, including the daily detox baths and complete adherence to the food list, for several months already? Have you completed Intro? Have you moved on to enjoy Full GAPS for several more months? Have you reviewed and addressed the common challenges presented within the previous chapter? If so, you will likely have found that many issues have resolved (if in doubt, refer back to the symptoms you recorded at the beginning of your journey, as suggested under *Months 1–3: Preparing for Full GAPS/Intro*).

Despite the gains to date, some symptoms may be persisting. At this point, you might choose to continue doing the program as is, allowing for the gentle healing to unfold in its time. However, if you have been doing GAPS for several months and you sense that further tweaks might enhance your healing, you might at this point consider some of the approaches that have worked well for people on our support lists. Experiment to find the best fits for you. The following list is presented in alphabetical order (not in order of helpfulness or any other criteria):

Antibiotics: If you continue to have problematic symptoms from *Klebsiella, Clostridium,* or another stubborn bacteria after six months of diligence on the GAPS program (including a therapeutic dose of probiotics), you might consider a course of antibiotics while otherwise adhering to the program. It will be critically important to continue the therapeutic dose of probiotics while taking antibiotics, but take these at a different time of day than you take the antibiotics.

Antifungals: The diet and detox aspects of the GAPS program will help to balance yeasts. Be sure to allow these aspects at least three months to do the initial work before deciding whether a next step is necessary—this can save you from an unnecessary degree of suffering (in compounding the die-off that you will already experience in early healing), as well as expense. Focus on diet, probiotics, kefir, and so on. If after the initial months of healing you intuit that a course of antifungals may be beneficial, there are several excellent options. In addition to the *S. boulardii* discussed later in this list, garlic, coconut oil, cloves, oil of oregano, and grapefruit seed extract are all very effective for reducing fungal overgrowths, including *Candida.* These products may trigger massive die-off. It is critical to incorporate just one at a time, starting with tiny doses and working up very slowly. Rotating them will prevent the fungi from adapting to them. I suggest starting with coconut oil, beginning with 5 mL (1 teaspoon) or less per day and working up slowly. When you can tolerate 15 mL (1 tablespoon), start using it regularly in raw dishes, such as in date-nut balls, in smoothies, or as a spread on baked goods. If more support is needed after a month of this, add *S. boulardii* to your program. I have also had success with the following protocol: one capsule (500 mg) of cloves each day for a week, then stop taking the cloves. The second week, take a single drop of oil of oregano each day then stop. The third week, take a single drop of grapefruit seed extract each day then stop. Begin the cycle again in the fourth week, but increase each product, in its turn, by one capsule or drop. In the seventh week, start the cycle again, but increase each product by another capsule or drop. After three cycles of progressive increases, take at least three weeks off. Some people require a more aggressive approach; they may need a prescription for Nystatin. (Other prescriptions may stave off the overgrowth while they are being taken, but the overgrowth will resurge when the prescription is stopped.) Pure bicarbonate of soda (baking soda) can be applied topically to fungal infections, or added to a bath (250 mL or 1 cup). On GAPS, baking soda is generally not to be ingested, but for balancing fungal infections (as well as for addressing heartburn), Dr. Campbell-McBride makes an exception and supports bicarbonate of soda being taken internally. In her FAQ document, she offers a recipe and instructions for this. You might also consider slowly introducing alkalinized drinking water into your program.

Blood sugar stabilizing: If mood or behaviour is an issue, be sure to apply the notes presented under *Health Issues: Hypoglycemia/Low Blood Sugar*.

Detoxifying baths: Do at least one daily, rotating the additive used (see *Detoxification: Die-Off Relief Baths*). Try to rest and/or sleep after a detox bath. During regressions or acute detox, consider having several of these baths daily.

Education: As a person of any age heals, he will become newly able to catch up on learning previously missed. This is not limited to academics, such as reading and math (although great gains will likely be made in these areas, too). Upon healing, each of us will hopefully have opportunities to learn anything we missed while our body focused on survival versus development. For a child, these new opportunities may be in areas such as speech, reading, movement, self-regulation, sleep habits, communication, or acceptance of a wider range of foods. In each of these areas special techniques and helpers exist; the Internet or your local child development centre can link you to options. Likewise, as a teenager or adult heals, she too will become vastly more capable of new approaches. Many things that people typically learn in a healthy childhood can be learned at a later stage, too. This may include any of the items listed above, as well as those in the areas of assertiveness, sociability, employment, boundaries, emotional self-care, and more. Healing allows relationships to be reinvigorated, new careers to be established, and a general enjoyment of life to be achieved. The support of a good counsellor, for example, can help a teenager or adult successfully transition, with their nutritional foundation in place, to a full life in which their dreams are finally realized.

Enemas (additional types): For people with specific healing needs, such as in cases of parasites, heavy metal overload, or chronic fatigue, Dr. Campbell-McBride suggests specific enema recipes. For details, please see Dr. Campbell-McBride's FAQ document. Within that document, do a search for all instances of your diagnosis or the word "enema."

Fasting: For people with more intense healing struggles, such as those dealing with fibromyalgia, Dr. Campbell-McBride suggests regular fasting. Specifically, one would nourish oneself well with marrow, soft tissues, and fats from the insides of animals, meats, and well-cooked vegetables for five days. On the fifth day, skip the evening meal, and take only water from that point for 24–36 hours, preferably enhancing this with water enemas to empty the bowels followed by a coffee enema to detoxify. Upon ending the fast, nourish yourself again with the abovementioned foods. For details on this process, please see Dr. Campbell-McBride's FAQ document, under "autoimmune."

Food combining: Your body may respond well to eating fruits (and preferably only local ones that have ripened on the plant) away from other foods (i.e., one hour before or two to three hours after any non-fruit). This allows complete digestion of each food and prevents fermentation in your gut. Conversely, your body may ask you to combine fruits with fermented foods (e.g., yogurt) or with fatty foods (e.g., nuts).

Heavy metal cleansing: If the tips listed under this Guide's section *Health Issues: Hypoglycemia/Low Blood Sugar* do not alleviate mood swings or behavioural issues, consider getting tested for an overload of heavy metals. If confirmed, treat as per the directions of your health care practitioner.

Intro: If you did not do the Intro progression early in your program, consider doing it now. Many people had so-so results until they did this. For those who did Intro early in their journey, returning to it occasionally can trigger a new depth of healing. At the time of this writing, I have done the GAPS' Intro progression a total of four times, each time to my clear benefit.

Juice only, until 10 AM: The body is in a detox cycle until approximately 10 AM. For some people, drinking only fresh, home-pressed juices until this time can greatly assist this process. At around 10 AM, proceed with a good GAPS breakfast.

Lifestyle changes: Diet can indeed make or break a person's well-being, but it is neither the cause of all issues nor a panacea. Once a foundation of healing has been set in place, it will be time to begin looking at other aspects of your life. Is your job totally misaligned with your soul's values? Did your child, pre-speech, learn to scream to get his needs met? Is your primary relationship a source of pain? Did your child become convinced that life is hard and that his way of being repels others? Have you been biting your nails for decades? Lives that have been distressed by nutritional imbalances for months or years may be impacted in many ways besides physically. We may have unconsciously established multiple survival techniques to get by during a period of suffering. These may have involved efforts to access nutrients (e.g., nail biting or binge eating); our means of communicating (e.g., screaming); or avoidance of activities, even pleasurable ones (e.g., work or spending time with friends). Stressful thoughts and behaviours can produce many internal toxins, which in themselves can interfere with our progress. With sufficient healing, old survival strategies are no longer required, but they may need to be specifically addressed in order to be replaced with more productive approaches, which we are now capable of. Counselling, behavioural consultation, career planning, meditation, Cognitive Behavioural Therapy (CBT), a move to a new location or job site, exercise, codependency therapy, etc., are among the approaches that may help us break behaviour patterns that no longer serve the new, healthier, better-functioning self. Many of these are offered without charge. Have faith in yourself and/or in your child. Know that you are ready to release the behaviours that helped when you were functioning in survival mode, and realize that you are now capable—due to your new physical, cognitive, and emotional resources—of new choices in communicating, working, and living. With a nutritional foundation in place, children often respond quickly to rewards of words or small toys, suddenly becoming able to move their bowels daily, or to communicate with calm, polite, cheerful words. An adult may quickly resolve chronic nail biting, for example, by wearing an elastic band around the wrist for a few days and snapping the band whenever the hand touches the mouth. Once diet has established a firm foundation of health, it is time to start looking at—not just through—the lenses of old perspectives, beliefs, patterns, and habits.

Oral infusion of probiotics: If thrush, oral sensitivity, mouthing, biting, or other mouth-centred issues persist, try this approach: After each meal and just before bed put a quarter of your daily dose of probiotic (homemade or commercial) onto your tongue and allow it to dissolve and rest in the mouth.

Organics: Switching to all-organic and/or pastured foods may bring increased results. Indeed, Dr. Campbell-McBride has found that some people's issues do not clear up until all pesticides and antibiotics have been removed from their diet. For tips on cutting the costs of these healthier options, please see *Practical Considerations: GAPS on a Budget.*

Organs: Many bodies do best when at least one serving of organ meat is included each week.

Parasite cleanse: Parasites are part of our lives and can exist in our bodies without necessarily causing problems. In the correct places in our bodies, they may even be helpful to us! Only in a compromised system or in cases of significant infestation will these cause noticeable issues. Thus, our primary focus should remain on getting the body deeply nourished and in balance. However, if healing is blocked, a parasite cleanse is worth considering. At one point during my GAPS program, I used Dr. Hulda Clark's protocol (http://www.drclark.net/en/cleanses_clean-ups/index.php) with great success. (I did not see parasites leave my body, but I did experience an increase in energy, a decrease in tongue coating, and—for the first time since childhood—my extreme nail biting stopped without any other intervention. Was this due to the antifungal action of the cloves, the removal of parasites, or another factor of the program? Without further and more methodical experimentation, I can't know.) Dr. Campbell-McBride recommends the allopathic drug, mebendazole. Each member of the household takes a 100 mg tablet twice a day for three days. Repeat this in two weeks and again every autumn (and more often if needed).

Reset the body: If you have come to rely too heavily on the texture of almond flour baked goods or on the sweetness of fruit and honey, consider resetting your habits and cravings by doing another round of Intro. Even three days on Stages 1–2 may be enough to redevelop an appreciation for the flavours, simplicity, and effects of a savoury diet. Alternatively, just remove your most relied-upon items from your diet until more optimal cravings and habits are established.

Review of Intro steps: Have you started to neglect any aspect of the Intro progression? For example, are you still eating lots of fats? Are you pouring olive oil onto every meal? Have you continued to eat at least 15 mL (1 tablespoon) of a ferment with every meal? Did you introduce your latest additions methodically? All of these are vital parts of the GAPS program, yet so easily forgotten! Review the Intro progression regularly and re-implement approaches that have inadvertently been dropped.

Rotate out foods: The strategy of removing one item at a time, as detailed in the *Food Issues: Food Sensitivities – Elimination and Reintroduction* section, is one method for pinpointing which foods may be interfering with healing. One member of a support list removed carrots and a persistent eczema disappeared!

Saccharomyces boulardii: This friendly yeast attacks and cleans up *Candida* and other pathogens. It is also useful in relieving diarrhea and, in some cases, constipation. It is very powerful and can trigger intense die-off! Be sure to start with a pinch of *S. boulardii*, working slowly up to the recommendations of the manufacturer or your health care practitioner, as die-off allows. In her FAQ document, Dr. Campbell-McBride provides her suggestions for dose and duration. NuTriVene (www.nutrivene.com) offers an excellent option for this supplement.

Seaweed: When all severe digestive symptoms have resolved, but a need for additional support is still indicated, Dr. Campbell-McBride has recommended to some clients to include seaweed. She notes that the Seagreens® brand is certified organic.

Supplements (other): For more ideas on supplements, see *Supplementation: Other Supplements.*

Vegetables: At various points in healing, including during hotter weather, you may find it beneficial to move from a richer diet to one including more vegetables, even up to 80% of your diet in volume. The math is not important; simply allow your body to guide you. Continue to include marrow, soft tissues, meats, animal fats, etc., but you might also enjoy a mixing bowl full of greens tossed with cubes of cheese and sauerkraut for breakfast, for example. As your body's needs change again—whether in response to internal needs or to cooler weather—it may ask you to return to the fattier, richer, protein-centred approach.

Water: The GAPS program inherently includes a lot of fluid with its broths, soups, whole vegetables, and fruits. Thus, the standard recommendation to "drink 1–2 litres of water each day" (which assumes one eats a Standard American Diet) is not necessarily fitting. This noted, increasing one's intake of water—preferably with a small amount of sea salt added, or in the form of another replenishing drink—can support the removal of toxins, relieve pain, and support bowel movements. Counting all your day's fluids, you might aim for 15 mL (0.5 fluid ounces) of liquid per pound of body weight. For example, a person who weighs 68 kg (150 pounds) might aim for 2250 mL (2.25 litres) or 75 fluid ounces (approximately 9 cups) of total fluids per day. Exercise, flu, die-off, ketosis, or ambient heat or aridity may increase the amount of fluid needed. So as not to interfere with the work of digestive juices, drink most liquids 30 minutes or more before (or 2½ hours after) meals. Avoid chugging water; rather, take it into your mouth then swish and "chew" it, allowing the digestion-supporting properties of your saliva to mix with it before swallowing.

Weight adjustments: As noted earlier in this Guide, GAPS—and especially Intro—will trigger an initial weight loss in most people and then a balancing. Underweight children and people who have been very thin (e.g., from Crohn's disease) will ultimately gain to a healthy weight. Overweight people will initially lose pounds. I had extra weight when I started, and over the first six months effortlessly lost 40 pounds. As long as I remain on strict GAPS, I hold steady at my ideal weight even while including the copious fats. When I experiment with non-GAPS food, my weight quickly increases.

After several months on GAPS, some may begin to see a slow, progressive gain beyond that which is healthy for them. If you are on strict GAPS and are ensuring that your diet is mostly marrow, soft tissues, fats from the insides of animals, meat, fish, eggs, organs, ferments, and vegetables (and very minimal in nuts, flours, and honey) yet you are gaining unnecessary weight, you may need to look at other triggers for weight gain. These include stress, lack of rest, disordered or insufficient sleep, hormonal imbalances, muscle loss resulting from insufficient protein intake or insufficient weight-bearing exercise (such as walking), physical stress brought on by too much exercise, or an excess of or a sensitivity to carbohydrates.

The importance of rest and sleep, the matter of how the physical stress of exercise can trigger an increase in body fat, and which types of exercise might be beneficial at various points in the healing journey are touched on in this Guide's sections *Months 1–3: Preparing for Full GAPS/Intro—Foundations for Healing* and *Health Issues: Exercise*. The matter of carbohydrates is more complex. According to Mark Sisson of *Primal Blueprint*, many people will lose weight if they ingest fewer than 100 grams of carbohydrates per day, maintain weight when ingesting 100–150 grams of carbohydrates per day, and slowly gain weight when ingesting more than 150 grams of carbohydrates per day. Decreasing or increasing carbohydrate intake (including over the amounts stated) according to your size, activity level, stage of healing, sensitivity to carbohydrates, and other factors may allow you to adjust your weight as needed for ultimate health and comfort. If you believe that carbohydrate sensitivity may be an issue for you, such that an undesirable degree of weight gain continues over many months even with lower amounts of carbohydrates, see this Guide's section *Food Issues: Assess Carbohydrate Sensitivity*.

For an overall understanding of the relationship between weight, carbohydrates, protein, muscle mass, energy, and other variables, I recommend the book *Curves: Permanent Results Without Permanent Dieting* by Gary Heavin and Carol Colman. Its "carbohydrate-sensitive" program is easily modified for GAPS. Additional excellent resources on this topic are the website and books by primal guru Mark Sisson (www.marksdailyapple.com).

...and Further

Additional options to consider include traditional sauna, the topical application of iodine, a daily dose of niacin, massage, swimming in salt water, mud baths, aromatherapy using certified therapeutic-grade essential oils, increased juicing, and homeopathy, among others.

For more details on any given approach mentioned anywhere within this Guide, and for additional ideas relevant to your specific symptom or body part of concern, ask your fellow support list members, do a search within the GAPSguide.com website, or do a search within Dr. Campbell-McBride's FAQ document.

As noted in this chapter, there is a lot of "wiggle room" within GAPS. Some of the ideas will work well for you and some will not. Any given person may need, for example, to remove apple cider vinegar; reduce their consumption of broth, fats, or salicylates; remove sweet vegetables; add liver; or include additional supplements. Aspects some people prioritize (but which I personally have not worried about) include the types of pots used, the quality of bath water, and so on. If these are a concern for you, they can be tested one at a time, just as a food might. That is, rotate out a type of cookware, chlorinated bath water, or any other item of concern, and watch for changes in your health upon excluding then reintroducing it.

Any given support, including any listed in this Guide, may or may not assist your particular body. Try out one at a time, giving each at least one month so you can see the results. Within the time frame that healing requires, there is plenty of room to try out different game plans. Go for it!

Finally, as you proceed through your healing journey, be sure to check the *Book Updates* page at the GAPSguide.com website at least monthly, as well as Dr. Campbell-McBride's regularly updated FAQ document.

CHAPTER 10
SPECIAL CONSIDERATIONS

GAPS Through Life's Stages

Note: For details of Dr. Campbell-McBride's recommendations regarding pregnancy, birthing, and beyond, be sure to read the expanded and revised edition of *Gut and Psychology Syndrome* (published in November 2010 or later), as well as any updates provided in Dr. Campbell-McBride's FAQ document.

Preconception

Ideally, the complete GAPS program—including the reduction of physical and emotional toxins in one's environment—is started many months before a baby's conception. If two people are planning a child, both would ideally go through GAPS' entire process (i.e., transitioning from one's current diet to Full GAPS, then Intro, then building back up to Full GAPS) before conception takes place. This provides the father with emotional centeredness and physical vigour as well as experience in shopping and meal preparation, so that he can fully support the mother. It allows the mother to approach pregnancy with strong physical and emotional reserves for an important and intense journey, not to mention peace of mind that she is doing everything possible to support her child through gestation. It ensures the baby receives the best possible material for the new human's basic building blocks, and maximum physical resources from which to develop. Granted, no dietary program can prevent every possible challenge or disability, and every human is gorgeous regardless of one's unique blueprint. Eating well before conception simply maximizes the resources that father, mother, and baby can access for the newest one's journey into this world.

Pregnancy and Baby's Early Days

If you didn't manage to do the full program before conceiving, fear not! The vast majority of people who come to GAPS do so during or after a child's gestation. Many of these babies get off to a good start in life regardless. Other children face distinct challenges, but the implementation of GAPS during their young years (or even adulthood) can bring excellent gains. Again, it is ideal to complete GAPS before conception—this is the simplest path to strong outcomes—but starting at other times also brings wonderful success, albeit with more effort involved.

If starting GAPS during pregnancy, it is recommended that you skip Intro and transition directly to Full GAPS. If you have not previously been using probiotic sources, including fermented foods, take special care with these in your pregnancy: start with a very tiny amount and work up slowly (see *Supplementation:*

Probiotics). Otherwise, include all aspects of the Full GAPS menu daily (minus anything you are reactive to). Eat the broth (either on its own or within a soup, stew, or casserole); the soft parts from in and around bones; meats; fish; liver and other organs; GAPS' fats with an emphasis on those from the inside of an animal; high-fat dairy (preferably raw and organic, if available) such as butter, kefir, sour cream, and aged cheeses; other fermented foods; and cod liver oil. Regularly include small oily fish such as mackerel, sardines, and herring. Ensure nuts are properly soaked (see *Recipes: More Essentials–Nuts and Seeds*). To avoid food reactions, Dr. Campbell-McBride recommends limiting raw fibre, opting most often for juiced or well-cooked vegetables and fruits. Juiced vegetables and fruits should be started with a very small amount and increased slowly. In her FAQ document, Dr. Campbell-McBride further recommends whisking a raw egg plus sour cream into your juices. Pregnant women with normal digestion who feel the need can enjoy small amounts of starches (e.g., potatoes, whole grains, and sourdough bread) if accompanied by copious fats.

Why not Intro? Doing Intro during pregnancy can potentially release the toxins from your system into the baby's system. It could also alter the nutritional composition of your milk. Finally, it could exacerbate the exhaustion common to many pregnancies. All of these are undesirable and almost always unnecessary.

Before receiving Dr. Campbell-McBride's directions regarding pregnancy, some women did do Intro during pregnancy. Even with these directions now in place, some women have opted to do Intro even while supporting another body directly, often because of severe allergies. Women doing so report mixed results: Some have reported that they felt too weak and tired to continue Intro while pregnant, and opted to move to Full GAPS as recommended; some have reported feeling well, clear, and strong with symptoms resolving in themselves, and strong babies being birthed. Your doctor, naturopath, or midwife can provide specific support if you are approaching GAPS while pregnant.

In the weeks leading up to the birth, prepare your birth canal and other areas of your body by smearing a handful of homemade yogurt or kefir all around your genital area, breasts, and armpits after every shower and bath. Let this dry before dressing. Dr. Campbell-McBride also recommends inserting beneficial probiotics into your vagina. For details and additional recommendations, please see her book *Gut and Psychology Syndrome*.

Caring for your baby inside and outside of your body will involve all GAPS protocols with the exception of Intro. That is, continue to reduce exposure to toxins such as chemical soaps, cleaners, air fresheners, chlorinated pools, cigarette smoke, perfume, and renovation materials as much as possible. At the same time, recognize that you cannot control every variable and that becoming overly stressed about toxins has its own negative impact on emotional and physical health. Just do what you can and remember that a body that is generally supported does have the capacity to process out a certain amount of unavoidable toxins.

Unless there has been specific exposure to a dangerous element, soaps are not generally necessary. Shampoos never are. Also, an approach called Elimination Communication (do an Internet search for details) supports a baby to go diaper-free. When diapers are used, cloth is preferable. Allowing your baby to roam at times without a diaper will allow her skin to breathe and rashes to heal. Any skin irritation can be soothed by applying coconut oil or homemade yogurt or kefir. Dr. Campbell-McBride recommends that a baby's mattress be wrapped in plastic, under the sheet, to prevent urine from mixing with microbes and chemicals contained within a mattress and potentially releasing toxic gases (Dr. Campbell-McBride believes this to be the main cause of crib death). For most of his life, my son and I have slept on folded blankets or simple mats on the floor. We find this very comfortable and the entire bed is machine washable! If new furniture is needed, more natural options can be researched. Ensure parents and baby enjoy daily, gentle walks in the fresh air, lots of rest, and as much relaxation as possible. Have plenty of support in place for the baby's first months, so that the mother can focus on rest and enjoyment and the father can focus on practical, emotional, and financial support of baby and mother. Friends, extended family, or hired help can take care of laundry, shopping, and more. Reducing exposure to chemicals is important, but the effects of love and joy must not be underestimated. Emotional and relational distress can cause a decline in health, while every increase in peace, connection, positive communication, receptivity, understanding, acceptance, and touch can make a massive difference in one's psychological and physical well-being.

Breast-Feeding

If you did not manage to do the full program before beginning to nurse a new baby, do not fret. For reassurance, please review the opening paragraph under *Pregnancy*.

If you are coming to GAPS with a young nursling in tow, you are likely doing so because you and/or the baby are struggling with symptoms. Even if just one of you is experiencing challenges, the inherent connection between mother and child means that the other likely has underlying issues; thus, it is best if both of you do the program.

If starting GAPS while breast-feeding, you will skip Intro and eat Full GAPS. For details on what to eat, please see the menu details offered under *Pregnancy and Baby's Early Days*. Doing Intro while breast-feeding has three potential adverse effects: (1) releasing the toxins from your system into the baby's; (2) changing the nutritional composition of your breast milk; and (3) reducing or ending your milk supply.

Several women did Intro during this stage of their baby's life before receiving Dr. Campbell-McBride's supplementary directions. I did, and both my son and I had only excellent results. In my case, though, my son was almost 3½ years old and had overcome his inability to eat the year before, so he was no longer entirely dependent on my breast milk. Thus, had my milk dried up, this would not have been too consequential. As it happened, my milk continued to flow until my son weaned himself a few months into our healing journey.

Even with Dr. Campbell-McBride's directions now in place, some women have opted to do Intro even while breast-feeding because of severe intolerances in themselves or their nurslings, for example. Some of these women have reported results similar to mine (i.e., they felt well, clear, and strong with symptoms resolving in themselves and/or their nurslings). Others have stated that their milk supply reduced or dried up upon starting Intro, and some reported that weakness and fatigue set in, prompting them to return to Full GAPS.

As a mother who nursed her child until he weaned himself at the age of 3½ years, I obviously support extended breast-feeding if that is nurturing for both child and mother. However, for the vast majority of children, I do not believe that nursing for so long is crucial. Full GAPS can well-support a baby nutritionally.

For mothers or babies having challenges with nursing that are not resolved through social supports, different techniques, or adaptive equipment, and the baby is not yet ready for solids, there are at least two options. One is to offer the baby milk from a healthy donor (preferably one eating a nutrient-dense diet herself), either directly as a wet nurse or indirectly through donations of breast milk to the baby's family. If this is unavailable, another option is to offer the baby a nutritionally sound, homemade formula. For recipe starting points, see The Weston A. Price Foundation website (www.westonaprice.org) or do an Internet search with a phrase such as "nutrient-dense baby formula." For babies who have reached at least four months of age, some parents simply add meat broth and other nutrient-dense foods to whatever formula is currently used and tolerated, and add additional puréed ingredients to the bottle over time until the infant is ready to transition to 100% GAPS foods in a bottle or on a spoon.

If considering doing Intro while breast-feeding, some things to reflect on include Dr. Campbell-McBride's recommendations, the age of your nursling (a baby under six months would be more affected by your milk drying up, whereas an older baby can thrive on Full GAPS without breast milk), and the degree to which any intolerances are causing problems in mother or child.

When intolerances are an issue for mother or child, but pregnancy or breast-feeding makes Intro less than ideal, consider the "elimination and reintroduction" strategy offered under *Food Issues: Food Sensitivities/Allergies*. The temporary removal of select foods is simple and safe. It does not provide the depth of healing that Intro does (which is why we should do Intro when it is appropriate to do so), but it can help identify intolerances and allow symptoms to be relieved without restricting the diet by more than one food (or food group) at a time.

Occasionally, dust or smear your nipples with a probiotic just before nursing (or before any other nuzzling if unable to nurse) so that your baby benefits from these. If your baby does not have an immunoglobulin E (IgE) allergy to dairy, you can also apply homemade whey or kefir to your armpits and breasts after bathing so that your infant can benefit additionally from contact with these areas.

With the information provided by Dr. Campbell-McBride in her book and FAQ document, your doctor, naturopath, or midwife can provide specific support to you if approaching GAPS in your baby's infancy.

Vaccinations

Many of the parents on our support lists did not have their children vaccinated, and many did. It seems that vaccination tipped the scales for some children, but that it was only one of many factors, as many unvaccinated children also suffer GAPS symptoms. In other words, complex health issues can develop whether or not one vaccinates; it all depends on the total toxic load. In her book *Gut and Psychology Syndrome,* Dr. Campbell-McBride offers a cautious approach to vaccinations that is specific to each person's medical history and state of health. Dr. Campbell-McBride suggests that a person not be vaccinated until they have developed a strong immune system and have good physical and communication skills (i.e., usually between three and five years of age). Dr. Campbell-McBride suggests that if a vaccine must be administered, that it be done while the child is in excellent health, that the list of ingredients be reviewed and considered by the parent, and that only one vaccination at a time be administered (with each at least three months apart from any other). Unfortunately, some countries offer combined vaccines only. Your pediatrician, family physician, naturopath, or osteopath can offer you information about options available in your area.

Baby's First Additional Foods

According to your baby's tolerances and with the guidance of your baby's health care provider, at approximately four to six months of age (when the baby indicates a desire to try solids), you may start to offer fatty broth, iron-rich organ meats (helpful from age six months on because the amount of iron in breast milk becomes too little to sustain a baby's iron needs after this point), meats in general, well-cooked vegetables, homemade whey, or the juice from home-fermented vegetables. Start with very small amounts, offering breast milk as a reward, and increasing the quantities over time.

To test for sensitivities and reactions, consider introducing just one new ingredient per week, removing any to which a reaction is obvious, leaving it out for a month or so, and then testing it again (except in the case of life-threatening reactions). Test a new food in the morning; if a reaction does occur, there are usually more resources available to us during the day.

As time goes on, introduce more and more GAPS foods. For many people—babies, children, and adults alike—any healthy food may need to be tried a good 20 times before we will really take to, enjoy, and desire it. Thus, offer your young one tiny amounts of any given food over the course of several weeks or months and allow time for her to adjust to it. Young children taught from the start to eat what the rest of the family is eating—their portion simply modified in texture or ingredients to prevent choking or other hazards—will be served both nutritionally and behaviourally, carving a path for many happy mealtimes for the whole family.

For parents who would like a very specific schedule for introducing foods to their baby, please see Dr. Campbell-McBride's book *Gut and Psychology Syndrome* (November 2010 edition).

Children

If dealing with a "picky eater," please also see the previous section, *Baby's First Additional Foods*, and also review the tips regarding eating broth, presented under *Recipes: More Essentials–Broth, Eating Broth*.

Generally, the younger a child is when introduced to GAPS, the easier the parents' (and child's) paths will be. Early in a child's life, the parent often has direct control over what food the child is near or offered, which can simplify things greatly. Having only stage-appropriate foods in the house and car means the child can graze freely without battle. Once a child is in daycare or school, or if he lives part-time with another parent who is not offering GAPS, he will be apt to stumble across non-GAPS foods. Depending on the circumstances, you have one or more of three options: (1) keep the situation unchanged and accept that the child may sometimes consume non-GAPS foods; (2) replace group daycare or school with a nanny or homelearning; or (3) help your child develop a personal commitment to the program so that he can do it in any location.

Of each of these options, only you know which ones are truly available to you. If the best that can be achieved is option (1), so be it! Consuming non-GAPS foods at times will, of course, slow the healing and likely bring on cycles of troublesome symptoms (although not more than a full-time diet of conventional foods will), but a good degree of healing can still happen. The child will also gain much healing simply in experiencing peace between parents who are separated but share custody, for example. In the meantime, your child will still be learning the value of true nutrition, practicing better habits that he can draw from in future efforts, and experiencing the effects of GAPS days and non-GAPS days. Allow the observational and learning capacities of your child to surprise you!

Many GAPS families choose homelearning. This gives full control of the diet to the parent, while the child can easily access nutritious food as soon as she is hungry. The child's homelearning curriculum can specifically include measuring, cooking, planning, nutrition, and so on.

As I am my son's only parent and we are dependent on my employment income, I have accessed different combinations of supports for my son over any given period of time: family members, conventional school (part-time and full-time), group childcare, and homelearning. In each of these situations, I chose adults who were able to honour my choices for my son. Also, for his first two years on GAPS, my son didn't blink an eye at our diet. When he finally started to express curiosity about the foods other kids were eating in preschool, I listened intently and developed new approaches (our experiences are reflected in the specific tips listed in the *Diet: What to Eat and When–Lunch* and *Practical Considerations: Holidays and Parties* sections of this Guide). I don't let dietary choices (mine or others') limit us from any activity; I simply plan more specifically and communicate more comprehensively with the other adults involved.

Older children, as well as some younger ones, may be fully able to commit to the program. Older children who understand the reasons for the program and its potential outcomes will often get fully on board and show complete commitment even when away from home. Do not underestimate a child's ability to comprehend the concepts involved, nor his desire to be as well as possible!

What about the child who cannot or will not eat? My own son was unable to eat anything but breast milk until after his second birthday. Except for on a handful of occasions, any other food—in some cases, even that which merely touched his lip—would cause him to vomit profusely. This was terrifying (not to mention physically draining for me because I was trying to breast-feed enough to sustain a large and active toddler). Except for very low iron levels, tests showed his nutritional profile to be strong. Doctors proposed having a feeding tube inserted out of concern for my own increasing weakness, but I declined, opting to continue breast-feeding. Eventually, my son became able to eat the vegetarian diet I was on at the time. He ultimately transitioned from that to the SCD then to GAPS.

My son's situation is becoming increasingly common, as are the following scenarios: children who eat only white food, food with sugary ketchup on it, processed foods, starchy foods (e.g., chips, potatoes, and rice), or very sweet foods; and children only able to consume liquid foods (e.g., breast milk, formula, intravenous therapy fluids, tube feedings, and meal replacement drinks) even after the age of three years. Children in all of these situations have successfully transitioned to the GAPS program and to excellent health.

Children, teens, and adults with an imbalance of gut flora are naturally repelled by wholesome foods. They are not being "picky," stubborn, or resistant. The pathogens in their guts are calling the shots. In their intense cravings for their preferred foods, the children can be like addicts, kicking and screaming if they don't get those foods on demand, and going through severe withdrawal symptoms when the foods are denied. Extreme responses to dietary limits or inclusions indicate that the body is off balance and requires resetting.

In this circumstance, what does one do? How does one transition such a child to the GAPS program? There are three options:

1. **Rewards:** You might offer your child one bite of his preferred food for every bite of a GAPS dish. Over time, make it one bite of the preferred food for every two, then three, then four bites of a GAPS dish. Feel free to start with GAPS cakes, pies, cookies, puddings, and other treats, especially those that offer the textures, fragrances, and temperatures preferred by your child. Non-food rewards that might help include movies, small toys, stickers on a chart, extra one-on-one time with daddy, and more. Even if this very slow, gentle approach is used initially, the two options presented subsequently may

ultimately be required to establish the child's capacity to eat the full range of GAPS foods.

2. **Transitioning:** In this approach, you will essentially follow the steps presented under *Months 1–3: Preparing for Full GAPS/Intro.* You will continue your child's normal diet while progressively adding in more and more GAPS foods until his whole diet is GAPS. Again, feel free to start with GAPS cakes, pies, cookies, puddings, and other treats. Children using bottles can have tiny, then increasingly larger, amounts of broth, etc., added to their usual fare. Use the same approach to offer the food on a spoon, then from a bowl, and so on. A child receiving his meals through a feeding tube during the night might test GAPS foods during the day and continue the tube feedings at night until the family, and their health care provider, is comfortable reducing or eliminating the tube feedings.

3. **Cold Turkey:** Some families have little time or energy to do either of the gradual approaches; other families are facing issues so severe that time is of the essence. These families might opt to go "cold turkey." In this approach, your child will be offered only GAPS foods from this point on. He may punch, scream, kick, and otherwise protest. He may decline all foods for up to five days. He may lose weight. All of this is fine as long as he stays hydrated (which demands not just water, but electrolytes). Whether he eats or not, he may be lethargic, weepy, and pale. He may vomit or have a fever. He may show any of the other symptoms listed under *Months 4–6: GAPS Intro Progression—What to Expect in Intro.* After a few days, he will begin accepting GAPS foods cheerfully and then want more and more. Parents are stunned to find their child ultimately free of cravings, with a fantastic appetite for meat, eggs, and vegetables. The child's spirit, skin, and energy will glow. Obviously, this is an incredibly difficult experience for a child or his parent to go through. However, it is so worth it!

If you are caring for a child with severe food limitations, do not begin any of the above processes until you have connected with the families on our online support lists, as well as with the health practitioner of your choice. Families who have successfully moved through these steps will be a crucial support in your journey! And by connecting with a practitioner before need is urgent, you will have someone available for immediate consultation if desired or required.

Children may also respond to any of the following:

• **Same food, different name.** A friend's daughter was initially repelled by a food called "beef," but would eat the same food when presented as "brown meat." Eventually, she became able to enjoy the food under any name (it turned out that she had overheard a beloved adult frequently voicing an aversion to beef and this had affected her willingness to try it). An omelette with cheese and veggies on top, instead of inside, may be accepted as "pizza." When my son was younger, he would readily accept blended and frozen savoury leftovers offered as "ice cream."

- **Participating in the preparation.** Many children feel more comfortable eating food when they feel in control of or know exactly what went into the dish.

- **Blending.** Many children, especially those struggling with texture issues, may eat a wider range of food when the dish is blended. Over time, you may be able to blend them less thoroughly, as new flavours are adjusted to and healing resolves the texture issues. So, instead of offering boiled chicken skin and soft parts as is or in a soup, perhaps blend them with some meat and herbs and offer the pâté as a dip, spread, or side dish. One child I know, who is not on GAPS, was willing to eat only a few foods, one of those being commercial pizza. Whenever I made a hearty beef-veggie sauce for zucchini noodles, I blended some to serve to him as "a bowl of pizza sauce." He loved it, and quickly became able to transition to the sauce unblended.

- **Find your "yes."** Determine an option you can say "yes" to and offer that. For example, my son loves to eat an apple, but he does best when all sugars are limited. Thus, each week I buy for him the smallest apple I can find. When he sees it in the house, he excitedly asks, "Can I have an apple?" And I can say "yes!" with ease.

- **Posted schedule.** When our children have visual "evidence" that more options are on their way, they often feel better about not having everything "right now." Before starting Intro, and as you move through it, show your child the Intro progression so that she can see that more is coming very shortly. (For a younger child, consider making a visual chart.) For my son, I also post on the fridge a list and schedule of snacks. It lists (1) all the foods he can choose from on any day without having to ask (e.g., two slices of cheese, raw veggies, leftovers, and boiled egg), (2) all the foods I'm willing to make for him at any time on his request (i.e., all forms of cooked eggs), and (3) for each day of the week, one additional special snack (e.g., banana, extra cheese, a high-quality pepperoni stick, or nut butter with honey mixed in). Every day of the week he is super excited about the special variation coming up and I'm free from questions, nagging, and constant negotiations. Some families include a "special snack" each week of a food advanced for the child's stage; provided this does not trigger obvious symptoms, this may be fine. Post-GAPS, I began including in my son's weekly rotation any non-GAPS food of his choice.

- **Novelty.** Many children enjoy a novelty approach, such as drinking soup (not too hot) through a straw, or eating from an insulated food container in a park. From a warm tube of bone freshly extracted from a soup, marrow can be sucked through a straw. While most of his meals are taken sitting in a chair at the dining table, I have noticed that my son will eat even food he's not currently keen on if it is offered "poolside" at his bath, or while he sits in a tree, or during a picnic on the sidewalk on the way home from his school.

- **Non-food rewards.** Many children will eat new foods when offered a reward such as a bike ride, a tiny new toy, or having an extra story read to them.

- **Choice where possible.** You will decide what food your child will be offered, but your child can still experience a great sense of empowerment by determining how much he will eat at any given meal or snack, what style of lunch kit to use, where to set up the family picnic, and so on. Allowing your child to make some of the choices that relate to his food will give him much peace and happiness.

- **Community.** Read to your child the stories of other children who have healed, such as the several offered within this book. On the e-mail support lists, ask if anyone has a child close to your child's age who would be willing to write yours a short letter of encouragement. Join or create a live support group so that your child can meet other children eating a GAPS, paleo, or WAPF diet, and attend potlucks where she can enjoy most or all of the dishes offered (the website www.meetup.com is an excellent resource for this).

- **GAPS Buffet.** When your child requests 15 bananas, is this a call for potassium or the result of spending an hour in a candy store and reminiscing about a pre-GAPS sugar rush? When caring for another person, how do we follow the body's lead? Just like adults, a child on GAPS quickly gains a healthy intuition regarding his needs. He may not, though, have the experience to identify the nature of his craving, the language to express it, or the research skills to look up which foods offer the same minerals. Thus, when my son has a hunger which my best efforts do not successfully satiate, I cover the dining room table with every food appropriate to the stage he's on.

It may include kefir, butter, seaweed, cooked meat, boiled eggs, an array of vegetables, and so on. If he is not experiencing an overwhelming craving for sugar, I trust that his body is in balance in this regard and I include a bit of fruit or almond flour baking. Over the course of an hour or two, he eats freely until he feels good again (he often chooses to eat butter by the tablespoon plus copious seaweed). His health, energy, and calm are excellent in the days following the buffet. In this way, I can support his intuitive awareness without having to spend endless effort guessing.

The voluntary eating of healthy food is a miracle that happens for another family within the GAPS community every week. Interestingly, we end up with the least fussy kids around. They are kids that eat vegetables while their peers gobble government-subsidized goldfish-shaped crackers. The best part is that you don't have to trick them: Once they're nourished, their bodies buy right in to the diet and they go full speed ahead.

One final thought specific to children: As my son got older, it became important to him emotionally to be able to keep any gifts of non-GAPS food he received. He doesn't necessarily feel the need to eat it—he just likes to keep what he receives, even if just to look at the package now and again. If I know I can trust myself not to dig into it, I let him keep it (but for my own sake I usually ask him to store it in a closed drawer). Because he collects a lot—sticks, goodie bags, free candies, and paper from school—every week we go through everything he owns and "release" anything extraneous. I choose how many things need to leave the house; he chooses which items will go. He often chooses to release each piece of junk food in favour of toys, notes from friends, etc. At times he is so taken by the form of junk food—a shiny wrapper or a toy attached to it—that he chooses to keep the candy. This is fine by me, as it helps him learn to be near candy without eating it, and how to recognize it for what it is: a non-food play item. This noted, after we transitioned off of GAPS, I began allowing him to eat up to one of these candies each week, and he has maintained a balanced approach to them (he seems to be more curious about them and keen on "being like other kids" than he is addicted to candy). When he indicates a stronger craving for candy, I know it's time to make him a fattier meal or to offer the buffet.

Youth

Depending on the age or needs of your youth, some of the information offered under the section *Children* will apply. Please review that and also consider the following.

Once a child is nine years of age or so, the family may be dealing with a different situation yet again. Your pre-teen or teenager may be very compliant, motivated, and self-disciplined. On the other hand, he may insist on a standard diet and disregard your concerns and best efforts. My personal opinion is that at this stage in your child's life, outside of a life-or-death situation or the potential need for the child's institutionalization, your hands may be somewhat tied. Your child may now be pursuing a strong degree of psychological independence and space, and he will also have increased access to money, stores, friend's houses, and so on. If your child is compliant or can be negotiated with, great! The GAPS community has indeed had several youth totally commit to the program, with excellent outcomes. If your child won't go for it, simply offer delicious GAPS meals at home and honour yourself and your youth by not fighting a losing battle. Instead, focus on making your GAPS meal times pleasant opportunities for connecting, show the effects of a nutrient-dense diet in your own life, occasionally mention youth-friendly benefits—such as joy, learning ability, clear skin, and a balanced body shape—and let your teen know that if ever she finds herself struggling mentally or physically, that you would be honoured to support her healing. During the challenges of young adulthood, many will feel unable to do GAPS 100%. However, having come from a home that recognized the value of true nutrition, your son or daughter will have sound information with which she can heal herself in adulthood, if she chooses. For inspiring accounts of youth who chose healing, please see the stories at the end of this book.

Adults

The challenge of GAPS in adulthood is that we are busy working and/or raising kids and/or finally "playing" (e.g., travelling) to the extent we dreamed of as kids! Also, socializing continues to revolve around food, and now alcohol is often added to the mix. Finally, we tend to put our children or career goals first, finding ourselves ravenous—or emotionally craving—at the end of each day, but too tired to prepare one more thing.

In terms of parenting, think of the oxygen mask analogy. Instructions on an airplane are: In case of flight failure, put on your own mask before placing one on your child. This is because we can only help our child if we are alive ourselves!

Because you are your patient as well as your own caregiver, you will need to ensure both roles are fully supported. Thus, whether you are doing GAPS just for yourself or while also supporting a child through it, make good use of the tips in this book for simplifying both your general lifestyle and your healing journey. Be sure to incorporate as much self-care as possible (e.g., a movie, a massage, a nap, counselling, and/or a non-food hobby such as scrapbooking or gardening).

Seniors

One reader asked me, "I'm 75. Is it even worth my doing the program?" My answer: "My grandmother is 95, still alive, and living independently. You may well have another 20 or more years to go! My wish for you is that all your years be as healthy as possible." GAPS can quickly alleviate symptoms of inflammation, pain, confusion, and more. The work of Dr. Abram Hoffer showed excellent results in alleviating symptoms of dementia, Alzheimer's, and similar profiles through dense nutrition plus vitamins. Personally, I would say it's worth a go.

Healthy Family Members

It is common for some family members to be healthier than others, thus I often receive the question: "My husband (or oldest child or another family member) is pretty healthy. I don't want to impose anything on him unnecessarily. Do you think he should do it, too?" If we take a closer look at this question, we see it implies that GAPS is a hardship. It's not. We need to be clear about this: GAPS is a healthy, nourishing, and satisfying program. People feel good on it. They enjoy it. Now, as to whether everyone in a family needs to adhere to it, here are my thoughts: Whether SCD, raw, vegetarian, traditional Cuban, or meat-and-potatoes, most families choose one eating program. Although not always a conscious decision, a choice is often made to continue the traditions of our family of origin, blend those with that of our partner's family of origin, or establish a new approach. Most families don't have as many food programs as there are family members. Every family makes a choice about what foods they're eating; inherently, each family imposes restrictions, even if only in terms of budget: "No son of mine is eating tofu!" or, "We always eat our quinoa with chickpeas. What else is there?!" or, "Sweetie, caviar is simply beyond our finances this week!"

When you choose GAPS, you are simply choosing one of the world's many menus. Choosing the "lowest common [dietary] denominator" is what works best for most families: it streamlines the shopping list, reduces meal preparation time, and supports everyone sitting together for mealtimes. Also, it is challenging to change habits, so if Dad continues drinking pop and nibbling on chips in front of the TV, it is going to be very hard for Junior to enjoy his vegetable sticks with almond dip. Healing requires support from family and friends. Clearly, I believe it is best for Dad to do it, too—at least in front of his partner and kids (he can always grab a non-GAPS snack when out of the house). Most fathers I'm aware of are very happy to support their children this way, as are most mothers, siblings, grandparents, etc., once they come to see the positive effects of the program.

Communicating with Others

The matter of diet can be as delicate a topic as religion or politics! I suggest limiting our statements and letting the results speak for themselves. As your child becomes calmer or more articulate, your skin becomes clearer, your child's school grades improve, and your iron levels stabilize, those around you will accept the power of your food choices. Most often, little if anything needs to be said. When we make strong verbal statements about our choices, those around us feel entitled to comment in response. Also, many of us feel vulnerable when we share the symptoms we're attempting to heal. Thus, I find a quieter approach generally more beneficial in our relationships, both with ourselves and with others. Absolutely advocate for your right to good food and to healing, but consider leaving it at that.

Some people really connect through food, and become frightened or hurt when opportunities for this are limited in any way. You can support others' desire to connect by actively inviting them to participate with you in activities that do not involve food. Bowling, kite flying, swimming, sun bathing, walking, conversing, and creating vision boards side-by-side are all great options! Alternatively, put out a GAPS spread and invite them for a feast.

Although people in our lives were supportive of our movement toward health, many of them were not able to understand how strictly I wanted my son and me to adhere to the program. When, upon their request, I provided them with a list of allowable foods, they were inclined to override it, either accidentally or because they assumed potatoes, for example, were "healthy" or "safe enough." Thus, I learned not to invite others to feed my son or me, and instead to say in advance of a visit something along the lines of: "We're following a temporary allergen-elimination diet, so we'll only be able to eat what we bring from home. We're excited to spend time with you, and my son will feel happiest if he's not offered additional foods. He will love receiving your affection and attention, though!" Some people will "make this about them" and take offense. At times, you will need to be quite strong, in terms of relational boundaries, in order to allow yourself (or your child) space to heal. A simple approach is to gently repeat yourself, as many times as necessary, until you are heard.

A note to your child's school or daycare might state simply: "My son is healing from multiple food sensitivities. During this intensive healing stage, please do not provide any food or drink except pure water and that sent from home." This approach, which indicates that the restrictions are temporary, alleviates the fear that many people have about a person's range of food being restricted, especially when it comes to foods they view as "healthy."

In person, when the topic comes up, cheerfully state: "We're following a temporary healing program recommended by a neurologist. The results have been amazing so far!" (Or, if just starting out, say, "A lot of families have had great results with it!") Then change the subject to the other person, inquiring about a non-food aspect of their life, such as their favourite hobby.

When someone offers unsolicited input, you might respond to the underlying concern with: "Thank you for that tip—I really appreciate you caring so much about me/my child." Again, subsequently change the subject to a topic that nourishes their own soul.

When preparing to host guests, explain: "We eat a diet recommended by a neurologist and nutritionist, and are seeing amazing results. We'd love to share our casseroles and soups with you. Would this work for you, or would you prefer to meet up after dinner?"

When preparing to be a guest, you might say: "We're eating a diet developed by a neurologist and nutritionist. As amazing as our results have been so far, we don't want our program to be any sort of burden on you. Would it work for you if we cooked for ourselves? If you're game, we'd love to feed you, too, in thanks for hosting us! Or would it work best for us to stop by after dinner [or have our meals out]?"

Upon receiving a gift of non-GAPS food, whether I've mentioned our diet before or not I find the best approach is to simply say, "Thank you!" In this phrase, I am responding to the thought and intention behind their offering, rather than to the item itself. I can subsequently pass the item along to someone who does eat that particular food. Before we see the person next, I make a point of casually mentioning, in person or in a letter: "By the way, we are now eating a diet prescribed by a neurologist. I won't be able to eat your lovely baking and homemade chocolates for a while! We're sure looking forward to our next hike with you, though. I'll bring some snacks to share with you!"

More and more physicians are becoming aware of the effects of nutrition, thus are becoming increasingly supportive of dietary interventions for a wide range of issues. Many GAPSters have had success finding a physician whose awareness encompasses biochemistry, the effects of nutrition, and similar or related fields. Others maintain a relationship with one physician for medical issues, such as an infection requiring antibiotic treatment, and enhance this with consultations with a second practitioner more focused on nutrition. I explain to physicians that we follow a program "developed by a neurologist who is also a nutritionist." This in itself doesn't seem to give them confidence in my approach, but the physicians I have chosen for my son and me do seem pleased when I respond to any of their concerns by volunteering to follow up with research, or with consultation with a dietitian, nutritionist, and so on (even a conventional dietitian is able to report to a physician the excellent levels of nutrition found in our diet). On the *Support for You* page at GAPSguide.com is a link to lists of health practitioners knowledgeable about dense nutrition, the experience of die-off, and all other aspects of the GAPS journey.

Be somewhat discreet, but not shy. Your choice for a healthy body need not be a source of shame, extended dialogue, or conflict. Remember: Each household chooses one general approach to food. No one has the right to criticize or control your choices. Brief, positive, cheerful statements should suffice.

Common Biases

"If all this is true, why don't they tell us?" Well, it depends who you mean by "they" because a psychiatrist, a neurologist, a nutritionist, and thousands of parents are telling you, and with much enthusiasm! Granted, not everyone is on board. Why not? Let's explore this…One sector often vilified on this count is the pharmaceutical industry. Although many people would express incredulity at this statement, the truth is there is a big place in my heart for these companies. Medications created by pharmaceutical companies may well have indirectly contributed to my original health issues, but they also ultimately saved my life. Their treatments helped me get to a place where I could start to explore true healing options. Bless them. However, their business is researching, promoting, and selling drug treatment options. I believe they want us all to be well, but they are definitely working from a different angle. They are not in the business of natural healing. They are in a different vein and a competing venture. Their passion is to develop and sell treatments, not to promote healing. Therefore, it's not their job to declare the wonders of asparagus.

"What about organizations dedicated to connecting their members with resources?" The fact that associations for people with celiac disease, Crohn's disease, autism, mental health issues, and so on rarely refer to or promote—and often actively discourage or dismiss—nutritional approaches is a source of immense frustration for those who have applied the program and who are

experiencing the best health of their lives as a result. Organizations tend to cite "studies" in which one or two foods or elements (e.g., gluten or casein) are eliminated from a diet for a few weeks, and no noticeable change occurs. Elements such as dyes, processed foods, and sugars remain in these diets, while nutrient-dense food, detox baths, and all other aspects of the synergistic GAPS program have no presence whatsoever. We could easily have anticipated for them zero results! A related argument against diet is that there are no double-blind studies proving the efficacy of GAPS, yet no one is offering to fund double-blind studies. Thus, patient testimonials (and personal medical charts, in some cases) are all we have.

Similarly, in the field of mental health, I read article after painful article declaring that diet has no impact on brain health or behaviour. Somehow, pills ingested do, but food ingested does not. Hmm…One otherwise lovely support worker once said to me, "Even if it worked, no one would stick with it." Defeatist beliefs like these leave suffering people to research, locate, and then implement these options in isolation. Also, mental health and social welfare systems frequently withhold services from those declining medication. Accordingly, a person in need of support must indicate that he is "in compliance" and not discuss diet. (In one hospital, my desire to do an elimination diet was viewed as an indication that I was unwell—it was categorized as an "eating disorder." Ironically, when I tried to access an eating disorder program for my extreme overconsumption of and binging on junk food, I was denied because this behaviour "does not meet the criteria of an eating disorder.")

I once witnessed the disability benefits appeal hearing of a severely depressed man who was terrified of taking medications. He was concerned about the impact of pharmaceuticals on his liver, as well as any potential for addiction to them. The appeal panel declared that because he was not taking medication, he was "clearly not very depressed" and that because he was concerned about possible addictive properties, he was "an addict." On these counts, he was denied funding for the nutrition that might otherwise have brought this very intelligent, earnest, and hardworking man to health.

There is also the dilemma that if one no longer has symptoms, she is often declared to have originally been misdiagnosed or "never actually ill" in the first place.

The abovementioned perspectives shed some light on why the SCD and GAPS are not yet promoted in the mainstream. But those of us finding recovery through them hold much faith that this will soon change.

Diagnoses—Multiple, Obtaining

"How would the same diet address symptoms of both celiac disease and autism, among other things?" First, we must note that both celiac disease and autism are challenging to diagnose. For example, there is a blood test that can tell you if you definitely have celiac disease, but the same test can't tell you that you don't. That is, if the test is negative, it doesn't mean you don't have celiac disease. Confusing? It gets worse. As with bipolar disorder, schizophrenia, anxiety, etc., autism cannot be determined by a pinprick or X ray. So, when anyone refers to autism, they are simply referring to a specific grouping of behaviours, many subjectively diagnosed. Bowel disorders tend to be variations on a theme, and "mental," neurological, or expressive differences are not much different. As such, a person with any of the above will often end up with several diagnoses, depending on who was doing the assessment and what the body happened to be up to within the relatively brief period of testing. The important thing to realize is that a person's gut doesn't care how many manifestations of the dysbiosis have been given a distinct name. An imbalanced gut affects mood, cognition, behaviour, blood sugar, mineral absorption, stools, and so on. You can call it "Crohn's disease and a really awful mood" or you can call it "chronic diarrhea and oh-by-the-way-he-has-screaming-fits-every-two-hours" or you can call it "autism with its typical constipation." My assertion is that in all such cases we're talking about one thing: an imbalance in the gut flora. It is commonly noted that (1) most kids with autism have chronic diarrhea, constipation, or both alternating, and (2) when bowel disorders are treated with the SCD, autistic symptoms clear. These symptoms dissolve regardless of whether or not a child has been labelled autistic. I'm not saying all kids with autism have celiac disease or that everyone with celiac disease also has autism. I'm saying that all these labels are nebulous and not as helpful as simply healing the gut is.

"Should I pursue a diagnosis before starting?" Your (or your child's) degree of suffering will answer that question. If you or your child are suffering deeply, you will likely be motivated to begin the program as soon as possible. Now, there is a specific advantage to being diagnosed first: funding (for more information, please see the section *Practical Considerations: GAPS on a Budget*). Because bowel disorders show themselves when under attack from specific foods and because "mental," neurological, and behavioural differences are diagnosed on the basis of current symptoms, doing the program will interfere with the diagnostic process. Without a firm diagnosis, any application for disability or nutritional benefits, as well as for occupational therapy and so on, is unlikely to be

approved. As GAPS is a relatively costly program, your finances may unfortunately demand that you pursue the diagnosis first. These noted, in terms of actual healing, a diagnosis doesn't matter one way or the other. Healing matters, and both diagnosed and undiagnosed people see results.

Other Diets

"I thought people with celiac disease just needed to avoid gluten." • *"How is GAPS different from the Specific Carbohydrate Diet?"* • *"Isn't meat a hard-to-digest food?"*

Different people recommend different diets. There is vegan, raw vegan, raw omnivorous, fruitarian, ovo-lacto-vegetarian, paleolithic, and others. Where does GAPS fit in? I believe that every program has potential benefits, and that different approaches will work best in our bodies at different times and under different circumstances. I am excited about the range of dietary options presented today, and more so about the healing each one has brought to different individuals. At the same time, I am aware that many find it confusing to determine whether to do GAPS or a different program. In this section, I discuss a few diets that I commonly receive questions about and explore these in relation to GAPS.

First, it should be noted that GAPS incorporates healing elements of many diets. It includes copious vegetables, supports the conscientious use of raw fish and raw dairy (if fermented), emphasizes beneficial bacterial and live enzymes, and incorporates juicing. A "paleolithic" diet is very similar to GAPS' early Intro stages. GAPS also has much in common with the diet advocated by The Weston A. Price Foundation.

In its synergistic approach, GAPS varies from other excellent diets in details that may make all the difference for an individual who is specifically pursuing the relief of severe bacterial imbalance. It removes many starches, emphasizes the use of broth, ferments, and other nutrient-dense foods, and incorporates an intensive healing progression (Intro), among other things. Of course, GAPS is not a panacea! One circumstance, for example, under which Dr. Campbell-McBride recommends a diet other than GAPS is in the case of cancer. For the healing of cancer, she recommends the Gerson Protocol, a strict vegan diet enhanced by juicing and coffee enemas. The Gerson Protocol is cleansing; the GAPS protocol includes cleansing elements, but it is equally focused on "building," which is critical to the issues GAPS aims to resolve.

Specific Carbohydrate Diet

The SCD is an excellent diet, successfully healing symptoms of Crohn's disease, autism, and more. In fact, the SCD is so good that it largely forms the dietary aspect of GAPS! What are the differences? There are a few. The SCD is specifically a diet, while GAPS is a three-part program: diet, detoxification, and supplementation. GAPS sets forth a different introductory protocol than that presented by the late Elaine Gottschall in her book, *Breaking the Vicious Cycle*. GAPS also relies more heavily on specific foods such as broth, kefir, vegetable ferments, and so on. While the SCD allows select store-bought juices, GAPS does not because pasteurization, additional ingredients, and potential for mould can all create significant challenges for GAPS patients (but homemade fruit and vegetable juices—full of nutrients and enzymes which help detoxify the body—are permitted and strongly encouraged). Elaine Gottschall had concerns about Bifidus and declared it "illegal" for the SCD. Dr. Campbell-McBride, on the other hand, actively supports the use of Bifidus. Finally, Dr. Campbell-McBride is less concerned about secondary ingredients, such as maltodextrin, used in a given supplement. Again, the SCD is an excellent diet and has brought and continues to bring incredible health to countless people. My son and I saw excellent results on the SCD, and additional ones on GAPS. Because the dietary aspect of GAPS is largely based on the SCD, many of us consider ourselves to be "members" of both communities.

Gluten-Free, Casein-Free

A gluten-free, casein-free (GFCF) diet does bring great relief to many people because it removes two major toxins from one's diet, but this addresses only part of the puzzle. Many people relying on the GFCF diet continue to incorporate heavily processed foods relatively low in nutrition and high in the carbohydrates that perpetuate the main issue: an imbalance of bacteria in the gut. GAPS goes well beyond the avoidance of two aggravating substances to actively heal the gut and deeply nourish the body.

The story of how a gluten-free diet came to be the accepted treatment for celiac disease is outlined in the book, *Breaking the Vicious Cycle*. Basically, the SCD was healing Crohn's disease, celiac disease, and more, but upon publication of a single paper, the gluten-free diet became more popular. Since then, it has been very difficult to get "competing" information out. For example, in its October 2008 edition, *Canadian Living* magazine published an article about celiac disease. It opened with the story of Jenny Lass, co-author of two SCD recipe books. The article somehow managed to forgo any mention of the SCD and discussed only gluten-free—even though Ms. Lass is gluten-free, lactose-free, and eats only the most digestible foods. Some people with celiac disease do great on the gluten-free diet; others have limited success. Those choosing it must stick with it permanently. Also, you will notice that many people doing GF tend to carry excess and disproportionate bulk around their middle, much like health-challenged people in the general population. Although their overall number of symptoms is reduced, this bulge is an indication of continued physical imbalance. A merely "gluten-free" diet can (and often does) maintain a dependence on processed foods and refined sugars, items that people with gut dysbiosis tend to heavily crave. The question, then, is whether a person aims to merely reduce symptoms or to reduce symptoms and achieve overall health. Those are two different goals, involving two different programs.

Vegetarian/Vegan

Many people coming to GAPS have been vegetarian or vegan for many years. Naturally, they struggle with the idea of including animal products in their diet. Other people considering GAPS are not necessarily vegetarian, but wonder if a diet free of animal products is the optimal route to health. Pre-GAPS, I had been vegetarian (or vegan at times) for most of 22 years (although during my pregnancies I did give in briefly to my sudden cravings for chicken). As my poor dietary history makes clear, my primary motivation regarding vegetarianism had always been animal welfare as opposed to personal health. When I learned about the SCD, I noticed that meat seemed to play a big role and this deterred me somewhat. However, my son was ill and I needed to do whatever it took to bring him to wellness, so I had to seriously consider this option. Because this matter is such an important one, I'd like to take a few paragraphs to delve into it.

Many health practitioners using diet to heal the gut recommend that meat be consumed for at least the first 6-8 weeks. This is largely because the introductory stage of any elimination diet would otherwise be too restricted. As gut healing allows for a wider variety of foods to be reintroduced, these practitioners advise that the quantity of meat can be progressively reduced, if desired.

Although Elaine Gottschall (SCD) used meat regularly, she indicated that the SCD could be done without flesh. But she stated that anyone attempting to do the SCD while also excluding eggs and/or dairy would have to research and implement additional steps to ensure their nutritional needs would be met.

Dr. Campbell-McBride does not make any suggestions one way or the other about the amount of meat consumed within the GAPS program. In fact, she notes that the amount and frequency of ingestion will be different for everyone. However, she does recommend that (1) children not be fed a vegan diet, and (2) a cup of meat broth—along with soft tissues, marrow, and fats from the inside of animals—should be consumed daily. Indeed, broth is one of the mainstays of the GAPS program—it has copious nutrients and also actively heals the gut lining. Dr. Campbell-McBride also notes that although plants are critical for cleansing the body (a very important aspect of GAPS), it is animal foods that build the body, including its detoxification system, and that raw animal products also assist in the detoxifying. Granted, animal products are said to carry a certain amount of toxins. This concept is frightening to people, especially for those already overloaded by toxins and for whom health is a goal. On this note, Dr. Campbell-McBride asks us to consider how many chemicals exist in other food sources as well: the ingestion of chemicals is unavoidable. Dr. Campbell-McBride proposes that in terms of chemicals (whether natural or synthetic) the best approach we can take is to actively build and support our detoxification system, feed it the cleanest sources of food we can access, and include a balance of building and cleansing foods in our diet. Thus, GAPS incorporates both animal and plant foods in whatever balance is optimal for each individual.

Some people worry that the consumption of meat or dairy is linked to cancer, eczema, or other ails. However, many people eat these over the course of their entire lifetime and do not develop these diseases. I believe that illness does not arise from a single variable, but that a wide range of factors are involved. GAPS does not include meat or dairy in standard forms nor in isolation; it includes specific forms of these within a program focused entirely on developing an efficient system for (1) digestion of nutrient-dense foods, and (2) detoxification. That is, it includes clean, properly prepared meat and dairy within the context of sufficient stomach acid, sufficient bacterial levels, appropriate levels of fats and ferments, and a diet free of processed foods and most starches. I believe these are the factors that most strongly determine health and resistance to illness.

All of the above considered, my personal conclusion is as follows: GAPS excludes soy, chick peas, grains, and other foods that many vegans rely on, and relies very much on meat broth, marrow, and gelatin for many nutritional elements, including calcium. Therefore, doing the program from the very beginning as a vegan would prove overly restricted.

Because my son and I could not initially tolerate eggs, dairy, or nuts, we did use meat daily for the first several weeks on GAPS. After about eight weeks, we were able to incorporate eggs from pastured chickens, and our intake of meat naturally dropped. A few months in, with nuts and seeds successfully introduced and summer's heat bearing down, my son and I went through a phase of eating only a small amount of wild fish about once a week. However, we were also using fish oil, fish liver oil, and meat broth. When winter set in, our consumption of meat increased again to two to three dishes weekly. Sometimes we eat meat (including fish) daily and sometimes we eat it just twice in a week, but it is a staple in our diet and clearly contributes to our well-being. (Ironically, we eat vastly more vegetables now than we did on our vegetarian diet.)

My sense is that without at least one of meat, dairy, or eggs, GAPS would be too restricted. Thus, my position is that GAPS with soft tissues, marrow, meat, and broth, but without dairy or eggs is fine; and GAPS with dairy, eggs, soft tissues, marrow, and broth, but without meat may also be fine. But GAPS without dairy, eggs, soft tissues, marrow, meat, and broth is not workable. A person committed to a diet entirely free of animal products should look for a different method of healing.

As far as I am aware, no one has yet developed and presented to the public a balanced vegan approach to healing the mind through the gut (if you know of one, I would sincerely like to hear about it because this is a common question and many committed vegetarians continue to suffer rather than do GAPS—it would be great if there were a program supporting this specific population). One vegan program is purported to heal bowel problems, but it does not offer any testimonials regarding cognitive or behavioural issues. That program is also permanent and even among the most devoted "natural hygienists" there is concern regarding permanent vegan diets, as well as veganism in children, such that even they recommend against it for anyone whose interest is health.

Again, a circumstance under which Dr. Campbell-McBride does recommend a vegan diet, and specifically as part of the Gerson Protocol, is in the case of cancer when a body needs to only cleanse (rather than build).

Finally, although I do now eat meat, I continue to care passionately about the treatment of animals. I do my very best to locate meats, fat, eggs, and dairy from animals that ranged freely and were treated as gently and conscientiously as possible throughout their lives.

Need for Proof

"I refuse to take on some extreme diet without proof, statistics, and references!"

The purpose of *GAPS Guide* is to share specific information and tips to ease the practical aspect of your journey. In this book, I have attempted to address the most commonly presented issues and questions that relate to implementing the program in a direct, concise manner. Because I am neither a researcher nor a health practitioner, my knowledge of "why" is limited. As a result, I am simply unable to answer questions like, "If some polysaccharides are allowed on GAPS, why aren't potatoes?" The truth is, I simply don't know and I have opted to invest my time and energy helping people with the practical aspects of a program which I have witnessed to have had profound healing effects in countless people rather than redirect my attention to the science. However, I respect that some people feel unable to commit to a program without having detailed information about why or how it works. Happily, much of the science is addressed in other resources!

Folks keen on the "why" or "how" of any aspect of the program are strongly encouraged to do one or more of the following: read Dr. Campbell-McBride's book *Gut and Psychology Syndrome* and the works cited in its bibliography, consult with Dr. Campbell-McBride or another health practitioner educated in the scientific aspects of the program, read Elaine Gottschall's book *Breaking the Vicious Cycle* and the works cited in its bibliography, or explore the additional resources linked to from the *Support for You* page at GAPSguide.com (look under the heading *Research*, where I link to a step-by-step guide devoted to helping you explore your questions).

In the meantime, personal testimonies about the effects of GAPS are available in countless e-mail list posts, blogs, and books.

CHAPTER 11
PRACTICAL CONSIDERATIONS

GAPS on a Budget

"Boxed macaroni and cheese is cheaper and basically all I can afford."

The financial impact of a nutrient-dense diet is one I know all too well. When I started the program, my income was extremely low. I rented out parts of my house and refinanced it three times in order to buy food (and to print the first edition of this book). I eventually released home ownership altogether. I'm very glad I did all of the above!

Unfortunately, much conventional food is heavily subsidized, while sustainably grown food is not.[1] The diet aspect of GAPS is more costly than a standard one—no two ways about it—but there are ways to reduce the bills. This is important, because many people coming to GAPS are on a very tight budget. Having kids with special needs, having special needs ourselves, and/or preparing all foods from scratch can interfere with our ability to work as many hours as we might otherwise. Further, whole, organic, and/or additive-free foods cost more than other foods. Finally, supplements can be expensive. Here are some tips to help you through:

- **Selecting From the List of Recommendations:** Recognize that GAPS is essentially a list of recommendations (e.g., supplements, amount of each supplement, and organic foods). The more of them you apply, the faster you may heal. However, leaving some out (e.g., the bottled probiotic, as at least one support list member has found) may still result in significant healing. You can also rotate in the various recommendations. For example, Dr. Campbell-McBride notes that some patients simply did not find significant healing until they switched to produce free of pesticides. This proved a key factor for those individuals. Although it is certainly desirable to limit the amount of synthetic chemicals entering one's body, this particular commitment is not necessary for everyone—many people have achieved excellent healing even while consuming non-organic food. Likewise, you may find that some of the healing recommendations are key for you and that others are not as critical. If your budget requires you to select and/or rotate in recommendations, invest primarily in the ones that are crucial for you.

- **"Clean" Veggies versus "Clean" Meats:** Dr. Campbell-McBride recommends that if your budget requires that you choose between organic

---

[1] For an exploration of this matter, see *The Omnivore's Dilemma* by Michael Pollan.

meats and organic vegetables, go with the organic vegetables (because vegetables do not have the inherent detoxification system that animals do).

- **Pesticide-Free versus Certified Organic:** Certification is an expensive process. Accordingly, many farmers who farm organically and/or otherwise sustainably simply do not have the certification. They may be offering organic produce at lower prices.

- **Local Farmers:** Local farmers often offer their goods at lower prices than stores do because they do not have to transport their goods long distances or divvy their profits with stores. Also, purchasing whole animals, or larger parts of animals, may save you a lot of money. Try farms, farmers' markets, and farmers' co-ops.

- **Grow Your Own:** If you have a balcony or yard, you can grow some of your own food. Focus on the more expensive produce, such as organic squash (which is very easy to grow). On a balcony, you can grow tomatoes, squash, cucumbers, and peas on trellises or in cylindrical wire containers. It's amazing what can be grown within a few square feet! In addition, many cities offer community gardens, in which individuals are provided with personal garden space within a city lot. Alternatively, a friend with a garden may be able to offer space. Finally, your landlord or a neighbour may be happy to offer a section of garden in trade for your help in keeping her yard maintained.

- **Price Checking:** Where I live, sunflower seeds cost one-fifth of the price of almonds or pecans. So, I use sunflower seeds far more often. Also, an organic butternut squash is $3 in season and $7 when out of season. Buy it in season, or check if the frozen version (if free of additives) is cheaper. Finally, a pot of celeriac costs me $13, but the same amount of cauliflower costs $4—both make an equally fantastic substitute for mashed potatoes.

- **Get More Bang for Your Buck:** For example, replace some meat with joints and bones from pastured animals: marrow-rich broth will supply deep nutrition and incredible flavour at minimal cost. Indeed, butchers will often offer bones, chicken backs, chicken feet, and chicken skins for next to nothing (you will still get plenty of protein from eggs, nuts, dairy, and certain vegetables).

- **Buy Online:** Because of lower overhead costs, businesses offering products online may be able to do so at significantly lower cost than those with storefronts can. Also, shipping on orders over a given amount is often free.

- **Stock Up:** When foods are in season, chop fruits and vegetables and freeze them. Tip: Lay the freshly cut pieces on a baking sheet and freeze them before moving the pieces into a freezer bag. This way, each frozen piece is separate from the next and you can grab just what you need, rather than having to thaw and use a whole block. When buying a large section of meat or a whole fish, you can ask your grocer to cut it into smaller parts for you and put it back into its bag (this service should be free). By freezing the meat in smaller parts, you can thaw and cook just one section at a time without having to pay a premium for buying each piece separately. Some members of our support list find a large freezer to be one of their best financial investments because it allows them to purchase entire sides of animals, for example, which significantly reduces the cost of each cut. In a small home, a freezer can be stored almost anywhere, even in a living room or bedroom.

- **Don't Stock Up:** Despite what I just said, bulk buying is not always a good idea! Specifically, don't stock up on any item you are still testing. If the item turns out to be a flop for your body, the cash is wasted. Limit bulk buying to items tried and true for you. Keep in mind, though, that what works for your body this month may not work for it next month!

- **Look for Used Appliances:** Internet lists like craigslist, Kijiji, and The Freecycle Network, plus local classifieds, can land you some items at excellent prices or even for free. Post a wanted ad, but also be sure to watch the "offered" posts (not everyone offering will bother looking through the "wanted" ads). Also try consignment and thrift shops, or even a note in a community newsletter. Finally, a member of a local GAPS, WAPF, or paleo group may be willing to loan you an appliance, such as a dehydrator or yogurt maker, or allow you to use theirs at their home.

- **Expanding the Food:** Soaking sunflower seeds, for example, almost doubles their volume. As a result, I'm paying half as much for my "pizza" crusts—and getting increased hydration to boot!

- **Use Everything:** When chopping vegetables, store any unused parts (e.g., peels and ends) in a bag in the freezer. Use these when you make a stock (strain them out after cooking). In our fridge this morning, leftovers from the past two days included poached salmon with skin, cooked cauliflower with ghee, cooked mushrooms and onions, and carrot mousse cake. I threw all of these together, blended them, formed the mass into patties and heated them in coconut oil. We happily enjoyed "burgers" for breakfast. If I had added an egg to the mix, the same combo would have been "pancakes." Blended but unheated, we would have eaten it as a "soufflé." Also, a whole animal is cheaper than the individual parts, and all of it can be used: From a whole chicken, for example, the skin, cartilage, etc., blended with some of the meat becomes a pâté. The bones can be used to create a healing broth.

- **Limit Expensive Foods:** My son and I generally eat whatever volume of fish is set before us, so if we cook a whole salmon, we eat a whole salmon. One day I realized how expensive that was, not to mention excessive. Currently, my son and I have nutritional need for only a handful of fish every week. If you, like us, eat whatever amount of an expensive dish is set before you, limit these in favour of lower-cost recipes such as stew.

- **Review Your Budget and Lifestyle:** Before starting GAPS and at least every year thereafter, revise your budget. Which is more important to you: cable television or health? Brand new CDs or balanced gut flora? A bedroom for each child, or vigour and happiness in each of them? Simply borrowing DVDs from the library instead of buying them might save your family enough to buy a high-quality fish oil. For some families, buying clothes at thrift stores can free up enough money to fund probiotics. With some organization, a bicycle, car co-op, or transit pass may meet your transportation needs and allow you to apply the costs of car maintenance, insurance, and fuel to your organic milk supplies. You get the idea. Sometimes, it's about finding money we already have.

- **Volunteer on a Farm:** An organization called *World Wide Opportunities on Organic Farms* (WWOOF) connects volunteers with organic farmers who need a hand. Labourers typically work about five hours per day and receive education and training plus free room and board (not to mention access to the health-enhancing elements of clean air, rich soil, gentle animals, and fresh-water swimming holes). Many WWOOF hosts eat a diet similar enough to GAPS that GAPS can be easily accommodated. Many farms accept entire families. Accommodations range from a tent site to a cabin or a room in the farmer's house. Your work may involve planting, harvesting, registering bed-and-breakfast guests, cleaning, caring for the farmer's children, or whatever agreement works for both you and your host.

- **Agencies, Government, and Service Clubs:** Third-party assistance may be available to you. Contact any agency in your community and ask for help locating funding for special dietary needs, books, and/or supplements. Note that funding is usually dependent on a firm diagnosis (see *Special Considerations: Diagnoses* and review *"Should I pursue a diagnosis before starting?"*). In British Columbia, Canada, for example, adults who require income assistance and have specific diagnoses can receive up to $40 per month toward special dietary needs. Further, adults who have a disability, very low income, and "wasting" symptoms may be eligible for up to $225 per month toward clean water, supplements, and special dietary approaches. Agencies may also be available to help you review your budget, free up hidden sources of cash, or locate subsidies for other areas of your life, allowing you to funnel more cash into healing. For example, if you are currently saving up to replace a leaky roof, Canada's Residential Rehabilitation Assistance Program may be able to cover that cost, freeing up cash for your family's dietary needs. (Sorry, I don't know what is available in other countries, but you get the idea!)

• **Transitional Funding:** Microlending is a community-based system that provides loans to people who are unable to obtain funding through more common routes, such as family or a bank. Individuals from throughout the world offer to loan a portion of the total amount required. When the full amount has been raised, it is transferred to the person in need. Although the interest rate (paid only to the agency facilitating the loan) can be high, a safe loan source can give a person the foothold needed to change her life (and to subsequently establish long-term, sufficient income). Lend4Health (http://lend4health.blogspot.ca/) facilitates interest-free microloans for the biomedical treatment of autism spectrum and related disorders. Kiva (www.kiva.org) allows field partner requests for "personal use" loans. If approved for a loan request, consider letting the GAPS community know via GAPSguide.com so that fellow GAPSters can chip in (I regularly loan through Kiva and would love to support your need this way). Finally, the Indiegogo website (www.indiegogo.com) allows anyone to request donations toward their personal or business goals.

Holidays and Parties

GAPS children and adults participate in every event of their choice. Wearing costumes, trick-or-treating, eating, dancing, eating, playing games, eating…Did I mention eating? Kids adjust very quickly to a special diet. They are so happy with the effects of true nutrition that they often don't care about the fact that everyone else is eating commercial crackers. Of course, you must be considerate of your child. For our structured parent/tot playgroup, I always brought a snack my son could eat. He took any ripe fruit from the shared plate, but also filled up on his own goodies while the other kids ate boxed cookies and commercial yogurt sticks. For our library's story time parties, the leader invited me to bring a special treat and put it on the group plate so that my son could be served just like all the other kids. For my son's fourth birthday, he was thrilled to be presented with his favourite pizza, a raw almond dish perfectly replicating the flavour and texture of refried beans, dipping veggies, and a big cake smothered in icing—all 100% GAPS-friendly!

Parents have come up with a variety of innovative ways to ensure that even Halloween and Easter can be fully enjoyed. Kids are happy as long as they are loved and nourished and get to enjoy fun foods regularly—they won't mind that they don't eat at McDonald's. Whatever the special event, approaches used by experienced GAPSters tend to follow some basic themes:

- If your child established any food traditions pre-GAPS, such as having a store-bought ice cream cake at every birthday, start talking with her about new ideas well before that event occurs next.

- Allow and support your child to participate in all aspects of a celebration, with the sole exception of eating junk food.

- Focus events on activities, rather than food. Instead of hunting for eggs or trick-or-treating, for example, spend the day making crafts based on the event's theme.

- Instead of relying on a candy hunt in your house or neighbourhood, find out whether your community is hosting any games, parties, or events specific to the occasion, but focused on activity versus food. In my region, popular community events at Easter or Halloween include treasure hunts, bobbing for apples, face painting, "haunted" house tours, visiting real bunnies and chicks at a petting zoo, or hunting for a plastic egg that can be traded for a small toy.

- Invite your child to gather up all loot offered, then follow through on one of the following agreements, as decided in advance:
  o You buy the loot from her (especially for an older child or teen), allowing her to spend the money as she wishes;
  o He puts the loot in a special place in your home or yard and "the candy fairy" replaces it during the night with a toy or cash;
  o The child trades the loot for a toy, half an hour to play his favourite computer game, or a trip to a swimming pool, etc.;

o   The child plays with the loot as a toy (my son loves to pretend lollipops are little people and creates a tiny puppet show with them);

o   Your child trades the loot for his favourite GAPS treat or meal; or

o   Your child collects the loot and then hands it back out to others with a special treat coming his way in the end.

For an Easter egg hunt, you can set out: plastic eggs that can be collected then traded for a toy of her choice; plastic eggs filled with tiny toys, stickers, or homemade date-nut rolls; a series of rhymes leading to a toy at the end; a bunny stuffy; or a wind-up hopping chick. One friend (whose children are not even on GAPS) invited his children to find eggs in a community hunt at a park and then re-hide them for other children. His five-year-old and eight-year-old were so excited to do this and to watch the other children finding them! My son once did a "reverse Halloween" where he gathered all the candies he had received at school into a basket and then took them door-to-door in our townhouse complex, handing the candies out to neighbours. The neighbours were delighted! Later, while my son enjoyed a GAPS treat at home, several of the neighbours brought my son gifts of fruit, toy cars, and stickers. In all the giving and receiving, my son's Halloween turned out to be a joyful, triple-round celebration of friendship!

For Halloween, sneak some GAPS-friendly treats into your child's bag for her to find and enjoy when she hands the rest over. Perhaps arrange for at least some neighbours to offer stickers, tiny toys, or fruit instead of candy. On one of the e-mail support lists, Catherine G. wrote: "Instead of collecting candy, we got a box from our favourite charity to collect money. We went door-to-door and told them we had food allergies but are collecting for charity any pennies they may have. In total we got $35; we are geeked about that. The boys were so excited to go out and help the poor; it was such a positive and uplifting night, filled with joy! At the end of the night they went to grandma's and got SCD-legal homemade candy. It was a blessed night. I highly recommend it. They get so excited when they get to pick out a charity that they have a personal interest in." For more inspiring, first-person accounts of what works for other families, start a discussion on one of the online support lists or search the GAPSguide.com website for terms like "Easter" and "Halloween."

For Jewish traditions, Elana Amsterdam offers on her blog (www.elanaspantry.com) a wealth of GAPS-friendly options. Do you have ideas about how your community's traditions might support GAPS? Let us know via GAPSguide.com!

Impatience

We are regularly encouraged to approach the program slowly and methodically. Despite seeing results from all of the other advice, many of us struggle to incorporate this one crucial suggestion.

Tell me about it! I was one who definitely had trouble implementing "slow and steady." I was a typical Type A personality: all about speed, very impulsive, and with virtually zero patience. Slow-and-steady superpowers came to me the hard way. Hopefully the following tips will make the path a little easier for you.

The Holy Grail is a Lot Less Shiny Now That I've Held It: Before starting GAPS, I had had five months' experience with the SCD, so I was familiar with the ultimate menu. As such, that menu no longer felt like a tempting "holy grail." A sense of "been there, done that" eliminates any sense of urgency for me.

The Gift of Screech: My first lapse in dietary vigilance made me very reluctant to experiment/cheat/jump again. My child screaming at me for five days and nights after a brief period of advanced and non-recommended foods left me feeling like I was just one more screech short of my own hospitalization. A very real trip to my doctor for coping drugs[1] was a hard lesson that I did not soon forget. Essentially, I developed "Posttraumatic Stress Disorder of SCD/GAPS Cheating." That did wonders for my "low and slow" motivation!

Satiation, oh, Blessed Satiation: From early on in GAPS, I was extremely satisfied with the thick soups. They provided flavour, simplicity, efficiency, and satisfaction such that I had never known! The thought of introducing more things was met by a sense of "ugh." I thought, "Why would I introduce something else? Then I would just have to spend more time cooking." Indeed, there has to be a really good reason for me to introduce more stuff when we are so content.

Vaccinating Against Reactions: When all else fails, logic bolsters my intention like nothing else. In my ongoing research, I stumbled across a tip based on the theory that "healthy foods heal." According to this theory, when a healthy, easily digested food causes problems, it is not necessarily because the food is a problem for the person, but rather that it may simply be triggering a healing crisis—same theory as with probiotics, right? That is, they are great for one's health, but starting with more than a tiny amount will likely lead to big reactions. This is also similar to the vaccine (especially homeopathic vaccine) theory. By starting with 5 mL (1 teaspoon) or less of a food, the body is triggered into healing, but without the crisis. The body gets to respond and adjust in its healing

---

[1] Ultimately I opted to put myself on SCD/GAPS, too, rather than use the pills.

process without freaking out. The "low and slow" approach to food introductions, detailed in the *Food Issues: Food Sensitivities/Allergies* section, can build tolerance of food that would otherwise be rejected by the body.

Limited Energy or Organization

No doubt about it, GAPS is more demanding than the Standard American Diet is. The first few months—as we move through the inherent lifestyle changes, a tremendous learning curve, and several rounds of die-off—are the most intense. As one person on our support list noted, "something's gotta give!" Managing in the long term is easier when the rest of one's life is in order. Here are some tips for simplifying so that good food can take over without everything else falling apart!

Prioritize

One of my favourite analogies for life goes something like this: Find a jar, a pile of pebbles sufficient to fill the jar, and three stones. Pour all the pebbles into the jar. When you subsequently try to add the three stones, you find there is no room left. But, if you first place the three stones into your empty jar, most or all of the pebbles will successfully fit in around those. The jar is our personal capacity. The stones represent the three or four most important aspects of our lives. The pebbles are "everything else." In approaching a program like GAPS, I propose that "excellent health" be a stone, not merely a pebble. That is, for the next 18–24 months, GAPS and just two or three other things (e.g., your personal spirituality, housing, time with your family, a volunteer gig close to your heart, or your career) are going to be your top priorities. The pebbles in your life might be conventional schooling, homeschooling, watching television, blogging or other hobbies, work when time off is an option, appeasing your in-laws, travel, and so on. For healing to occur, it is critical to make your program a priority. Review your priorities annually to achieve the life that is most effective for you.

Efficiency

- **Be where you're at.** After your initial read of this entire Guide and Dr. Campbell-McBride's FAQ document, refuse to read about anything that doesn't pertain to your life today. Thus, while you are on Stage 3 of GAPS, attend to only those posts, recipes, articles, and tips about Stage 3.

- **Take time.** I am only truly effective in solitude and silence. So, before my son was in mainstream school, I paid my sister to take care of my son for five hours a day, six days of the week while I worked, cooked, and did self-care. This is what made GAPS possible for me (consider that no one expects a person to be able to pull off construction or office work with little ones underfoot!). If you have a spouse, ask him or her to take the kids out for at least two hours each day. Can a friend, relative, neighbour, or professional support person stay with them for another hour or two? If these are not an option and you cannot fully function with the kids at home, consider placing a child in daycare or in school, if currently homelearning. Although homeschooling is an ideal for many GAPS parents, one might reconsider the mainstream option for at least the first year or two on GAPS. Conversely, if having your kids at home is not problematic, and your region's laws allow it, you might opt for "unschooling," a movement in which a child's learning is supported by natural participation in all of life. (Although my own GAPS issues forced me to drop out of high school, by making my health a priority I was able to eventually attend university, where I came in at the top of my classes. I was not harmed by the time off.) Similarly, people who are working or in school might take vacation days or even a year-long sabbatical in order to support their healing. GAPS is relatively time- and labour-intensive; you need to free up some space.

- **Unplug the TV.** Put the television in an inconvenient place so that you can still watch a particular show if you really want to, but it will demand enough effort that you will think twice about setting aside your precious time for this. Also, consider quitting the news altogether. Except perhaps for emergency weather alerts, most news is unnecessary, not to mention a big drain on emotional energy, which can also directly impact healing.

- **Calculate.** I speak from personal experience when I say that do-it-yourselfers tend to get very overwhelmed. Often, it is cheaper and faster to let someone else do stuff for you. Unless it is vital that you learn this specific skill at this specific time in your life, don't do it. Maybe you don't have to learn how to make fermented vegetables this week. And maybe you don't have to make your own diapers. If you could save $20 doing it yourself, but it would take you four hours to do, it may be more effective to take a contract paying $5.50 per hour and then buy a given product (or pay someone else a little bit less to make it for you).

- **Commune.** In the Community Kitchens program, folks interested in similar dishes meet regularly to cook up a storm. After just three to four hours, each takes home numerous freezable portions for their family. An alternative to this formal approach is to invite a friend over once a week to push shredded cabbage into your respective jars, chop veggies into sealable containers, or simmer a vat of soup to share.

Getting Help

- **Teach.** Depending on their ages and with a little guidance the first few times, children can run a juicer, run a blender, mix, put nuts to soak, sauté, chop veggies, or find recipes. Back to the topic of homeschooling, this all counts! Meal preparation teaches nutrition, math, science, and organization, not to mention one of the most vital life skills!

- **Delegate.** While you focus your hours on learning GAPS, a spouse or older child can manage the laundry, dishwashing, tidying, cleaning, and so on.

Food

- **Prepare just one menu for the household.** Even conventional wisdom recommends that the family chef not become a short-order cook. GAPS is nourishing for all. If the family dynamic requires it, allow non-GAPSters to simply add potatoes or bread as a side to their GAPS meal. This is already plenty of compromise; more may simply exhaust you (see the section *Special Considerations: Healthy Family Members*).

- **Prepare only one major meal per day.** There is no need to spend your life in the kitchen. If you are most energetic upon waking, use that time to prepare a large batch of one main dish, such as stew, chili, soup, or a casserole. Eat this for breakfast, fill an insulated food container for lunch, and refrigerate the rest for supper or a subsequent day's meal. (In this aspect, Intro is actually one of the simplest times we experience on GAPS!) Throughout the day, enjoy leftovers from any previous meal, or grab-and-go items such as a glass of kefir, quickly scrambled eggs, a whole cucumber, a handful of nuts, a piece of cheese, or a whole bell pepper eaten in the same way as a whole apple. GAPS does not need to be three different from-scratch meals per day!

- **Use simple recipes.** Some folks really enjoy a gourmet approach to GAPS, but if you are like me and you prefer recipes that involve no more than three steps, options abound! On the GAPSguide.com website are lots of ideas plus links to many simple recipes.

- **Recycle recipes.** Keep a folder of your five simplest dinner recipes, or a binder listing simple breakfast, lunch, supper, and snack ideas. When overwhelmed, use one of these meal options.

- **Create a master shopping list.** Develop a list of your staple foods and supplies based on your current stage of GAPS and personal tolerances and preferences. As you move through the program, modify it as needed. Once a week, print off your list, walk through your house and cross off anything you have enough of for the week. Shop for everything that is not crossed off. By using this method, you do not have to make shopping lists from scratch and you always have all desired ingredients on hand!

De-Clutter

- **Reduce.** One of the easiest ways to relieve overwhelm is to get rid of anything you don't need. This can include a relationship with a person who is draining your energy, a volunteer position on a board, the excess mugs that just create a larger dish load, or a car when walking or transit is an option. To start: Set a container into one corner of your house. Every time you notice something around your home that you don't want or need, simply drop it into the container. When it's full, ask a thrift shop or a freecycler (www.freecycle.org) to pick up the contents. If you have extra time and energy, you might choose to sell some items on craigslist or Kijiji to gather funds for GAPS food and tools. I have been very surprised to find that my son is far happier with fewer toys than more! Same goes for me. For more tips on reducing, see the *Simplifying* category on the GAPSguide.com website.

- **Put it in its place…almost.** Move all household members' personal items out of common areas daily and set them into each one's respective room or bin. Let them decide what to do with the stuff from there. This frees up the kitchen for food work.

- **Take it outside.** I love doing crafts, but I don't want to fill my home with clutter. My solution? I organize craft sessions at a local church, seniors' centre, or playgroup. They provide the space, pay for and store the supplies, and do the major cleaning, while I have an hour of blissful activity and make the world a happier place for those who join me! When the session is over, I walk away and return to my nice, clean home.

- **Prevent.** You can call your postal service and ask them to stop delivering all flyers and bulk mail to your home, for example. Who needs the extra job of sorting through, reviewing, and recycling unsolicited materials?

Downsize

- **Move.** Although this may sound drastic, this worked wonders for me. In the house I lived in when I started GAPS, I was in over my head. The space was far more than I needed, demanded a lot of maintenance, cost too much, and was restricting my life in more ways than I even realized! When a small, low-cost rental came up, I jumped at the chance (even though I was scared). Wow! That was the best decision I could have made. My second GAPS home involved no extraneous work. I have since made four more moves, each time to a smaller, cheaper, lower-maintenance space. Wherever I am, my home isn't fancy—it is small, modest, and simple—but it really frees up time and money for healing, which is definitely a priority for me.

Limited Time

My primary food shortcut is to make one very simple meal each day. I don't fuss, I don't go for gourmet, and I aim to prepare in a single pot. Many mornings, I simply cook onions and sole in a pot, add salt, serve it for breakfast, and fill our insulated food containers with it for lunch. I may do the same with scrambled eggs or omelettes. If I have a bit more time, I might grate a cauliflower into onions sautéed with ground beef, adding in chili and curry powder. The following are some additional options for making your GAPS program simpler and faster.

Meal Plans: Through the *Support for You* page at GAPSguide.com, you can find meal plans made by experienced GAPSters. These go beyond recipes to offer day-by-day menus. While most cost a nominal fee, the time and energy saved may be well worth it! Available at the time of this writing are meal plans relevant to every stage of Intro, Full GAPS, dairy-free GAPS, egg-free GAPS, and more.

Re-evaluating Your Approaches: For example, in the *Recipes: Ferments* section of this Guide, you will find one very detailed kefir-making guide and one very brief one. I used the steps set out in the extended version until I was familiar enough with the process that I could set aside some of the proscribed steps and wing my own approach. As time goes on, you will develop in all aspects of your program your own processes, menus, patterns, and habits. Do allow those. When we first approach GAPS, we're experiencing a huge learning curve and often the wisest thing to do is to follow directions exactly as laid out for maximum efficiency and results. Once we have some healing under our belt and understand the general concepts and goals of any given aspect, we can start playing a bit and develop approaches that best suit our preferred lifestyle.

Commercially Prepared Foods: Using commercially prepared or processed foods can be challenging. For one, not all countries require all of the ingredients used in processing or in the final product to be listed on the packaging. This noted, after several months of healing, you might decide it is worth the effort to contact companies to learn which ones use only GAPS ingredients and allow yourself to use those on occasion. Indeed, more and more companies are offering very integral foods, including encapsulated raw organs, cultured vegetables, and more. In some cases, making our own is the cheapest option; having quality foods carefully prepared for us may come at some expense. But the time and energy that is freed up may make it worth investing in prepared items occasionally. Recently, I've been picking up a hot, cooked, whole chicken (flavoured with just spices) from a local health food store once a week. My son and I eat some of the meat immediately, save some to have as snacks or in stir-fry over the subsequent day or two, then simmer the bones in our next soup or broth.

At the time of writing, Organic World in Canada (http://organic-world.ca/) and U.S. Wellness Meats in the United States (www.grasslandbeef.com) are good online resources for quality meat cuts. I trust there are countless others. Companies such as Digestive Wellness (www.digestivewellness.com) and JK Gourmet (www.jkgourmet.com) offer delivery of SCD-compliant flours, baked goods, portable treats, and more. Dr. Ron's Ultra-Pure (www.drrons.com) offers quality organs freeze-dried and encapsulated. A number of companies offer live fermented vegetables—ask your local health food store what brands they carry. LÄRABARs (www.larabar.com) are popular amongst GAPSters, but be aware that some of their newest flavours have undesirable ingredients added in. Old-school butchers are popping up in more and more regions to provide not only additive-free meats as unique as buffalo, but also marrow bones cut horizontally and duck fat by the litre.

Please note that except for those intentionally creating options compliant with SCD and/or GAPS, a company's ingredients and processes are subject to change. With any prepared food, ensure alignment with GAPS by giving ongoing attention to food labels or through regular communication with the company about its manufacturing processes.

Eating Out: With sufficient healing, you may find your body able to tolerate foods prepared at restaurants, which may or may not have small amounts of non-GAPS ingredients incorporated. An increasing number of restaurants and coffee shops are offering options specific to GAPS, WAPF, and paleo diets, but choices extend also to Mongolian grill buffets, steakhouses, traditional Vietnamese menus (simply decline the noodles and rice), or any establishment which allows one to order a plain meat patty, a slab of roast, or grilled fish alongside plain greens. At a food court, order "sides" of meat and greens for a complete GAPS meal. A popular international coffee shop chain now offers organic dried mangoes, whole bananas, and nuts with no added ingredients. All of this noted, except for at WAPF/GAPS/paleo restaurants, or those you otherwise know to use only quality ingredients, limit restaurant meals because many will use poor quality ingredients, such as processed oils that are hard on the body regardless of whether or not the meal contains specific non-GAPS ingredients.

In short, while it is entirely possible to do GAPS completely "from scratch," supportive options are increasing and these can allow you a break now and then. My hope is that every region of the world will have at least one person start a blog listing GAPS resources available in that area. (Have you done so? Let me know so I can list your webpage on the *Support for You* page at GAPSguide.com!)

Spirituality

Every spiritual or religious community has its own traditions. These may include practices such as fasting, feasting, taking communion, or abstaining from certain foods. For many people, spirituality is a key element to their overall well-being, and GAPS need not interfere with this at all. Following are some ideas to consider.

If your community practices communion with bread, ask your minister for a blessing instead. If receiving the communion bread is very important to you, release any worry about this particular exception to the protocol (the healing that results from a spiritual practice may well override the effects of any small physical variation to the program). Alternatively, consider choosing the gluten-free option often offered. Although still a starch, it may have less impact on your body than a gluten-inclusive one might.

If your tradition includes periods of fasting, consider scheduling Intro during a non-fasting time of the year. Intro can trigger tremendous healing, which in many people requires the support of very frequent meals. Outside of Intro, GAPS can absolutely honour fasting practices.

When feasting is implemented, simply plan ahead for a GAPS version. Elana Amsterdam provides on her blog (www.elanaspantry.com) entire menu plans for Jewish celebrations; the vast majority of ingredients she uses are GAPS-friendly and the few that are not can easily be substituted.

In terms of abstaining from specific foods, such as pork or an item not prepared in a specific way, note that any item on the list of recommended foods can be omitted from one's personal program.

GAPS supports all people, the world over.

CHAPTER 12

HEALTH ISSUES

"But besides Candida, I also have chronic fatigue syndrome and fibromyalgia. Should I treat those first?" • *"I've done GAPS for six weeks now and I'm still struggling. I think my adrenals are shot."* • *"I can't digest the amount of fat included in this program!"*

Most people coming to GAPS present lengthy lists of health problems, including fat malabsorption issues, compromised thyroid and adrenals, and more. Most will find that symptoms of any chronic health problem—regardless of the name that issue has been given—are resolved through the program without special modifications. Again, the premise of GAPS is that the gut is your body's control panel (i.e., it determines how all of your body's systems are functioning). GAPS as presented is intended to address all the manifestations of gut dysbiosis, but some health concerns may be most supported by emphasizing specific aspects of GAPS or by including complementary therapies right from the start, as detailed in the following sections.

Addiction

A number of GAPSters have faced some form of harmful dependence, whether on processed food, alcohol, prescription or non-prescription drugs, cutting, binging, purging, or another item or activity. Regardless of the form the addiction takes, a multi-faceted approach is critical. Sobriety will reduce much of the internal and relational impact that intoxication or self-injury can create, but folks also report that dense nutrition makes all the difference in their capacity to become or remain substance-free, as well as in how well they feel while abstaining. Some have been surprised to find they spontaneously gave up an addictive substance or behaviour within days of starting an allergen-free and/or nutrient-dense diet. Others had already committed to sobriety, but continued to struggle with depression, anxiety, low self-esteem, confusion, and more (all of which can put one at risk of establishing or resuming an addiction) until implementing deep nutrition. Because GAPS resolves these persistent symptoms in many people, it dovetails beautifully with addiction-recovery programs.

One key to addiction recovery is to maintain stable blood sugar levels. Please be sure to follow the directions provided under *Hypoglycemia/Low Blood Sugar* as well as the rest of the material provided in this section.

If any GAPS food triggers a craving for your substance or behaviour of concern, keep it out of your diet. Some people with addiction to alcohol, for example, choose to keep vanilla out of their home and diet. It is absolutely fine to do so. (So far, people with an addiction to alcohol have reported that fermented foods—such as apple cider vinegar, sauerkraut, and kefir—have not triggered their addiction.)

Be sure to include all tolerated GAPS supplements. The oils, for example, may prove critical for keeping moods stable and cravings curbed. When symptoms or cravings persist, consider consulting with one of the supports listed in this Guide's section, *Supplementation: Other Supplements*. The work of the late Dr. Hoffer, for example, has been beneficial for many who had previously struggled with addiction. Bill W., co-founder of the Alcoholics Anonymous program, was firmly committed to abstinence from alcohol as well as to spirituality and peer support. Despite this, he continued to experience significant depression and fatigue. After many years of sobriety, Bill W. was introduced to Dr. Hoffer's nutritional therapy, and implemented the niacin aspect of it immediately. He experienced profound relief from the symptoms that had plagued him for so long. Bill W. subsequently wrote about his experience, and expended much effort to share the impact of this treatment with the world.[1]

Supports such as counselling, eye movement desensitization and reprocessing (EMDR), and/or a 12-Step program can help one decline the addictive substance and to implement self-care (including GAPS). Although 12-Step programs tend to consider nutrition an adjunct therapy and do not allow it to be promoted within meetings, it can certainly be implemented privately while one continues to access meetings for peer support in abstinence. Further, the Overeaters Anonymous program (www.oa.org) can be implemented by choosing GAPS as your nutritional protocol and having your program support you to stick with GAPS 100%, as opposed to counting or limiting calories, fats, or portion sizes.

At the time of this writing, the only addiction-specific GAPS resource is a section on GAPSguide.com. However, several people committed to their sobriety are connecting there and keeping each other and new contacts supported. I strongly encourage anyone needing support in finding or maintaining sobriety to connect with others through the website and through the GAPS e-mail lists. All are linked to from the *Support for You* page on the GAPSguide.com website.

Adrenals

Follow the general GAPS guidelines, while also ensuring you are taking in lots of fat and cholesterol (e.g., animal fats, egg yolks, sour cream, butter, and fatty fish). Sufficient rest—much more than people without adrenal issues may require—is

---

[1] See http://vitaminb-3therapy.blogspot.ca/

critical. A low-stress perspective (as opposed to simply a low-stress lifestyle) is also key. Approaches such as Cognitive Behavioural Therapy or EMDR can make all the difference. Some GAPSters have been well-served by natural adrenal supplements prescribed by their health care practitioner. Again, I recommend most people allow the GAPS program, including Intro, a full three to six months to support the body before assessing whether an adjunct therapy is required, but this will ultimately be a decision between you and your health care provider.

Bloating or Gas

Gas or bloating may be caused by any of the following:

- Probiotics (as a supplement or fermented food);
- Yeast overgrowth or yeast activity;
- Die-off (whether from diet, probiotics, or an antifungal);
- Low digestive juices;
- Menses; and/or
- Inability to digest a particular food.

It is very difficult (read: basically impossible) to know for certain the cause of any given round of gas or bloating. This section is intended to help you narrow it down. Regardless of the cause of bloating, while it persists, continue the healing progression as presented, modified by the following additional tips.

Probiotics (including fermented foods): If gas or bloating occurred shortly after introducing or increasing one's dose of fermented vegetables, fermented dairy, or bottled probiotics, it is reasonably safe to assume this is the cause. Decrease the dose and rebuild more slowly (see the *Supplementation: Probiotics* section of this Guide). Note that Dr. Campbell-McBride recommends that fermented vegetables be started with just 5 mL (1 teaspoon) per day of the juice only. Once increased juices are well tolerated, only then should one begin with 5 mL (1 teaspoon) of the fermented vegetable itself and work up from there.

Yeast activity or overgrowth: When bloating persists even after all other die-off symptoms disappear, the issue may be due to yeast overgrowth, where an imbalance no longer needed to serve the body is still in the process of being reduced. Conversely, it may be required yeast activity, in which yeasts are attempting active cleanup of other toxins, such as heavy metals. For yeast overgrowth not specific to other "jobs," general yeast-reduction strategies may help (see *Health Issues: Candida Overgrowth*). When yeast is actively working to address more serious issues, its by-products (e.g., gas and bloating) will likely persist despite specific efforts to reduce them. Again, true healing is methodical and requires some patience. Allow your body to do its work. After at least three months of implementing the general program, Intro, and the tips under *Health Issues: Candida Overgrowth*, review the tips provided by Dr. Campbell-McBride in her FAQ document. Namely, consider implementing the tips she presents there for incorporating heavy metal cleansers, such as those mentioned in this Guide's *Detoxification: Juicing* section, and the use of garlic enemas.

Die-off: For tips to avoid or decrease gas or bloating (and other symptoms) from die-off, see the section of this Guide *Relief from Transitional Discomfort*.

Low digestive juices: Gas or bloating may be caused by low digestive juices. Please apply the tips listed under *Health Issues: Heartburn, Reflux, and Indigestion*.

Menses: If triggered by menses, bloating should subside a few days after menstruation begins. This issue should eventually resolve altogether on GAPS. Some *Candida* specialists suggest increasing doses of yeast killers for one week before one's period is expected to begin.

Inability to digest a new food: If you develop gas or bloating upon adding a new food, your body may not yet be able to tolerate that new food. Follow the tips under the *Food Issues: Food Sensitivities/Allergies* section.

Digestive enzymes: People challenged by bloating which persists despite all of the previous tips may be well-served by a course of supplemental digestive enzymes. Test these at the dose prescribed by their manufacturer and, after another month on continued GAPS, start reducing the dose by a small amount every week or so. If the bloating resumes, return to and maintain the immediately previous dose for another month.

If none of these helps and you have been diligent about the program, consider the items listed under the section *Progressing Further*, such as a parasite cleanse.

Candida Overgrowth

Many people come to GAPS struggling over the question of whether to implement an anti-*Candida* diet or GAPS. Struggle no more! For most people, GAPS as presented heals an overgrowth of *Candida*—a yeast that is a healthy and necessary part of our internal ecosystem, but which can trigger frustrating symptoms when overgrown. The GAPS program as presented—especially with short-term adherence to early Intro—addresses this, just as it does numerous other imbalances. That is, many people will experience dramatically reduced *Candida* numbers even while eating moderate amounts of GAPS' honey, fruits, sugary veggies, and nuts as complements to the program's primary foods. Early in my SCD/GAPS journey, I completed a self-test for *Candida* overgrowth.

Distributed by Yeast Buster, the questionnaire invited me to assign a score to each of a long list of symptoms. A total of 80 points indicates a "severe" overgrowth. I initially scored a whopping 200. Within eight weeks of starting the SCD, my numbers had dropped to 25 (indicating that overgrowth was unlikely at that point)—I was indeed feeling very well.

If after a few months on the program—including a round of Intro and all of GAPS' daily detoxification steps, such as daily bowel movements—you intuit that a more aggressive approach is required, you might opt to limit or avoid GAPS' fruit, honey, and sweet vegetables. (It will not be possible, or necessary, to completely avoid all sources of sugars, so don't worry about minute amounts in foods or supplements.) In terms of the vegetables, this means removing beets, carrots, orange-fleshed squashes (e.g., butternut), and sweet onions. Copious vegetables and fruits continue to be available to you, most of which can be eaten well-cooked, raw, or anywhere in between. These include French artichoke, asparagus, avocado, bok choy, broccoli, Brussels sprouts, cabbage, cauliflower, celeriac, celery, collard greens, cucumber, eggplant, garlic, ginger root, kale, lettuce, mushrooms, yellow (i.e., not "sweet") onions, parsley, peas, bell peppers, spinach, non-sweet squash (e.g., spaghetti), string beans, tomatoes, watercress, and zucchini.

Probiotics, and the friendly yeasts in kefir, will also do wonders. These will be critical to introduce. The natural antifungal properties of coconut oil, starting with 5 mL (1 teaspoon) and working up slowly, can also have profound effects.

After all of these have been incorporated for at least three months, you might also consider implementing a course of *S. boulardii*, a friendly yeast that knocks out then mops the floor with *Candida* (see the *Progressing Further* section of this Guide).

If oral thrush persists, after each meal and just before bed put a quarter of your daily dose of probiotic (homemade or powder) onto your tongue and allow it to dissolve and rest in the mouth.

Finally, be sure to check Dr. Campbell-McBride's FAQ document for additional tips. If further support is required, see this Guide's section *Progressing Further* for additional antifungal options and more.

CFS and Fibromyalgia

Conditions such as chronic fatigue syndrome (CFS), also known as myalgic encephalomyelitis (ME), and fibromyalgia indicate that the breakdown of the body has reached a deep degree. Healing may require more time and patience than other manifestations of gut imbalance might. In addition to the regular GAPS program, consider the following.

First, approach yourself as a "sensitive or very ill" person, following the recommendations within this Guide for the gentlest approach to GAPS. Thus, your transition to GAPS may be closer to 12 weeks than 4 weeks, your starting dose of probiotics will be the lowest amount indicated—or even less—and you will give yourself even more rest than most people on GAPS will require. A detox bath before a nap or nighttime sleep may prove very supportive. Dr. Campbell-McBride recommends that you skip the foods that are challenging for you, while adding in those that are better tolerated even earlier than otherwise suggested. Dr. Campbell-McBride also suggests that betaine HCL with pepsin at the beginning of a meal and pancreatic enzymes at the end of a meal may be of benefit to you. Finally, Dr. Campbell-McBride suggests eating meats, fats, and well-cooked vegetables for five days, then fasting on water for 24–36 hours (preferably enhancing this with a coffee enema) before repeating this cycle. For details, please see Dr. Campbell-McBride's FAQ document.

Second, after a few months on the program, you may want to consider incorporating other therapies for healing and retraining the mind's habituated processes, which greatly impact your body's physical ones. One option for this is Gupta Amygdala Retraining (GAR). Components of the GAR program, such as Neuro-Linguistic Programming (NLP) and/or Cognitive Behavioural Therapy (CBT) may prove very helpful even on their own.

Cravings and Hunger

"I can't live without rice cakes." • *"But I don't feel full unless I finish my meal with bread!"* • *"I can do GAPS if I can eat fruit every day; I just can't live without it!"*

Before the SCD, I consumed Twinkies, chips, candies, chocolate bars, and a bottle of pop almost every day. Did I say "and"? Yes, all of them, almost every day! It was how I kept going, how I kept my energy up, and how I coped. Because I had given these up before, I knew it was possible to do so again, but I could not fathom how. Plus, I felt discouraged about trying again because every time I had given them up, I had eventually taken them up again. Additionally, each time I had eliminated them from my diet, I had faced difficulties: cravings, fatigue, and the uncovering of bizarre health problems. On GAPS, these concerns proved unfounded. From the first day, I had little to no cravings—and no strange symptoms were unmasked this time!

It is critical to recognize that until you stop eating all non-GAPS foods and sufficiently nourish yourself with GAPS foods, you will continue to have intense cravings for non-GAPS foods or foods too advanced for your stage of healing. It is also very common to believe we cannot feel full unless we eat bread or pasta. Neither of these situations indicates that you "need carbs" (e.g., grains). Rather, most cravings—especially persistent ones for excess sweets (including fruit) and breads—indicate the need for a reset (see *Progressing Further*).

Cravings will disappear when you are well-nourished. In the beginning, becoming well-nourished involves eating a tremendous amount of food, in as wide a variety as possible, and as often as the body indicates need. For most people, this means eating marrow, protein (e.g., meat or eggs), and fat plus any other stage-friendly GAPS food upon waking, at least every hour or two throughout the day, and again right before bed. This increased need to eat is temporary; it will balance out (usually within 6 weeks or so). In the meantime, avoiding or limiting nourishment will leave one hungry, shaky, depressed, and wanting foods outside of one's current stage. After the initial transition comes to a close, the need to eat so much and so often naturally subsides. Ultimately, most people thrive on just two to three meals and one to two snacks per day.

Taking fat regularly, as recommended previously, often eliminates a craving for sugar. In this vein, Dr. Campbell-McBride's tip for a portable blood sugar stabilizer will also be helpful (see *Health Issues: Hypoglycemia/Low Blood Sugar*).

Another effective approach to cravings is to find out which key minerals are associated with the desired food and to choose a GAPS food that contains those. A simple Internet search will tell us that cocoa, for example, offers a good dose of magnesium. Early GAPS foods rich in magnesium include Swiss chard, spinach, pumpkin seeds, green beans, halibut, almonds, mineral water, and more. Eating these foods may end the craving for the non-GAPS food and actually leave us feeling even better than our go-to food (e.g., a chocolate bar) would have! In fact, during early Intro, magnesium supplementation in the form of whole foods, juiced produce, or commercial powder is helpful for many to end cravings, and it can also relieve tremors, insomnia, leg cramps, and constipation.

To prevent and manage cravings, it is critical that you feed yourself as needed and that you do not attempt to limit the frequency or amount of healthy foods. GAPS nourishes you. We may have previously established a habit of eating junk food to provide us with energy, a feeling of satiation, or a sense of calm. Whole foods taken regularly and in abundance provide these benefits without any of the processed food's side effects.

Eczema

Eczema is an issue for many people coming to GAPS. Some people hit on their personal solution quite early on and find relief within days. For others, this symptom is far more stubborn. Its resolution is much slower in coming, and terrible flares are experienced in the interim. However, on our support list we have seen decades-long persistent eczema resolve in mere days, weeks, or months. (I had a form of eczema that an international specialist in the natural healing of skin conditions said could only be healed by wearing gloves during all daily activities for six months. Happily, the following faster remedies did the trick.)

Eczema is often linked to a compromised gut, thus it can be exacerbated in any healing crisis or die-off. Therefore, the management of die-off is critically important in this situation. Eczema may also require additional attention—and even exceptions to the GAPS protocol in some cases. I suggest the following approaches, in the order presented.

While healing is taking place on its own schedule, these remedies can be used to soothe and calm the skin. Please note that what works for each person is different; a remedy that works for one person may exacerbate symptoms in another. It is a matter of trial and error.

1. **Urgent Care:** For some people, eczema will resolve upon even a single dietary change, such as removing wheat or dairy. For others, resolving eczema can take more time. In the meantime, it is important to stop the cycle of thinned skin, scratching, and sleeplessness. Give irritated skin a chance to heal through the following steps:

    • Ensure the humidity level of your home is at a healthy level, and that it is not too dry.

    • Avoid environmental triggers. Make sure you are not using chemicals, even those found in sunscreens or in some "natural" laundry detergents, such as ammonium lauryl sulphate. Wear cotton clothing. Avoid feather pillows. Clean your bedding regularly so that dust and mites do not exacerbate it. Wash clothes and bedding regularly in hot soapy water.

    • Reduce the temperature, frequency, and duration of any showers or baths. Even die-off relief (detox) baths may need to be limited for a while. In any bath you do have, be sure to use one of the die-off relief bath additives. Rotate them to see which soothe the eczema, which make it worse, and which make no difference. Continue using those that soothe or do not exacerbate the eczema. If all baths and showers exacerbate the eczema and must be avoided, achieve the benefits of a die-off relief bath via a foot soak.

- After washing, pat—do not rub—the skin dry, then apply ghee, butter, shea butter, olive oil, cocoa butter, or another rich food to the affected skin (coconut oil may also be useful, but may also increase one's internal die-off). Slather the affected body part and then cover it (with the exception of one's face, of course) with plastic wrap or cotton clothes—including socks or gloves—and leave overnight. For some, a topical application of honey, avocado, or probiotic powder mixed into avocado helps.

- Increase your intake of dietary fats and/or liquids.

- In cases of intolerable itch or an itch that results in intense scratching, temporary use of a natural remedy or even a commercial lotion may be helpful in hydrating and strengthening compromised skin long enough to end an itch cycle and allow the body to adjust and heal through dietary approaches. The Aveeno® line of products made specifically for very dry skin and eczema, including the oatmeal bath, is one that might be well tolerated. It is preferable to avoid cortisone or other topical corticosteroids, but their temporary use may be necessary in extreme cases. If you are actively scratching, keep your nails very short to allow healing to complete.

2. **Basic Healing**

- As noted throughout this Guide, a daily bowel movement is critical to allow toxins to exit the body. Ensure at least one—and preferably up to three—bowel movements daily. Use an enema if necessary.

- Proceed slowly. Desperate for relief, many people leap into multiple healing practices early on. This can cause fast and horrendous die-off, including exacerbated eczema, pus, and blisters. Stopping or slowing supplements, antifungal foods, all probiotic sources, etc., can ease the die-off. Although it is probably the most difficult thing to do on GAPS, moving very slowly and methodically can make all the difference and allow healing to happen at a manageable pace.

- For some people, the addition of probiotics (e.g., yogurt, fermented vegetables, or commercial capsules) resolves this symptom. For others, the same thing triggers a flare-up, but this is not always as negative as it seems. Although intensely uncomfortable, a flare-up often indicates that intense healing is taking place, and can precede a full and permanent resolution of the symptom. To minimize the issues and maximize the benefits associated with taking a probiotic, follow the recommendations in the *Supplementation: Probiotics* section of this Guide, especially in terms of starting with a tiny amount and working up very slowly.

- Be sure to do the Intro progression and then work methodically through the program.

- Include copious GAPS fats.

- If you know or suspect that a specific food is triggering the eczema, remove it. The problematic foods are different for everyone. To determine what foods may be an issue for you, and when and how to retest or reintroduce them, follow the steps offered within this Guide's section *Food Issues: Food Sensitivities/Allergies*. Some foods or groups known to trigger eczema in different people within the GAPS community include one or more of: fermented vegetables, sweet foods (including orange vegetables and/or fruit), nightshades (e.g., tomatoes, bell peppers, and eggplant), dairy, legumes, foods containing higher amounts of oxalates, and non-GAPS foods such as grains. As noted in the section *Food Issues: Food Sensitivities/Allergies*, one of the simplest ways to determine which foods trigger a reaction in you is to start with a very simple Intro and add new foods one at a time while observing reactions. Elimination and reintroduction of a suspected food at any other point in your program, as detailed in that section, can also be very helpful.

- Chiropractic adjustment, deep tissue massage, and similar approaches have resolved eczema in many, often in as little as one treatment.

- On the GAPSguide.com website, I maintain a page dedicated to the symptom of eczema. Check that post and its comments for specific remedies that have worked for some members of our community.

3. **Advanced Steps.** If eczema is still present after a complete transition to GAPS, a full round of Intro, several subsequent months on Full GAPS, and application of all of the previously mentioned tips, it may be time to consider more intensive healing support. Again, advanced remedies can be too much for a severely compromised system, triggering an unbearable degree of eczema that is also more difficult to resolve. In most cases, it is best to provide the body with a good foundation before proceeding with these.

Advanced treatments may be antifungal, anti-parasite, or liver cleansing, among others. For ideas, see this Guide's section *Progressing Further*. Remember: A slow, gentle approach to healing is often as effective as a fast and intense one, with less pain.

4. **Hang In there!** Eczema can be very stubborn. It may flare and diminish multiple times over the course of healing. Seasonal allergies, which may take one or two seasons to fully heal, can exacerbate eczema that has been otherwise lying low. Do not be discouraged by flare-ups.

Exercise

GAPS is an excellent program for people keen on developing their fitness capacity. The healing of conditions such as chronic fatigue or asthma clears the path for a person wishing to incorporate more movement. People committed to fitness before coming to GAPS find that the fats provide an excellent source of energy, while the protein supports the building and repair of muscle. With dense nutrition, one's overall energy, endurance, and recovery time increase. Long distance runners and aerobics instructors are among those doing GAPS successfully. When they are hungry, they increase their fats.

Although GAPS can support fitness, is exercise always a good thing? When I was a patient in various psychiatric care facilities, I was repeatedly given the very firm message that regular exercise would heal anxiety and lift depression. For me, it didn't. For me, it exacerbated both. Running, weights…any intensive movement would rapidly deplete me, leaving me even more jittery, despondent, and lethargic than I had been an hour before, and struggling even harder to recover "emotionally." When I finally declined the hospitals' message and listened to the one my own body was giving me instead, my journey eased significantly. Brendan Brazier, a professional triathlete and health trainer who advocates a low-grain vegan diet, strongly believes in exercise, but even he sets forth important caveats. In his excellent book, *The Thrive Diet: The Whole Food Way to Losing Weight, Reducing Stress, and Staying Healthy for Life*, Brazier notes that any form of stress, including exercise, can set hormones off balance, which in turn can cause weight gain. Overriding one's need for rest in favour of physical exertion, or working out when the body actually needs an opportunity to build its nutritional reserves, can cause vulnerable people to gain weight in the form of fat, especially around the belly. If you struggle with fatigue or other health symptoms, and are actively pursuing a healing program such as GAPS, allow yourself a lot of rest. Move your body only when your body (and not your adrenaline addiction) requests it. When your energy is up, just enjoy it, or move your body more. As you heal, your energy will increase and you will naturally gravitate toward movement, starting with gentle options and moving progressively toward more intensive ones, as the body desires.

GAPSters have done well starting with just rest for many months, then moving to options such as gentle stretching to music, yoga, walks, gardening, and housework. Over time, your capacity will increase, and you will be able to incorporate hiking in nature; playing with your children (e.g., hopscotch, skipping, monkey bars, etc.); cycling; swimming in non-chlorinated water; a core-strengthening program, such as Pilates; an uplifting movement program, such as Nia; or a gentle strength-training program. For the latter, you might use just your own body weight (e.g., push-ups), incorporate wearable weights (e.g., ankle weights while walking), or access hydraulic machines, such as those offered by Curves International (www.curves.com). Even gentle resistance can build muscles for overall health, comfort, energy, posture, and weight loss or maintenance.

As your health increases even further, your body will let you know when you are ready to seek deeper exercise. At that point, a great resource is the online community organized by Mark Sisson (www.marksdailyapple.com), which primarily advocates short stints of vigorous "play." Personally, I love participating in a Meetup group (www.meetup.com) devoted to all variations of the childhood game of tag. We move quickly and intensely, rest as needed, laugh a lot, and are outdoors in sun, rain, or snow. (I have noticed that I play—and recover—distinctly better when I've been doing GAPS 100% for at least one week leading up to it.)

In summary, exercise is a positive thing when it grounds an anxious state; begets more calm, happiness, and physical energy; leads to a good sleep; and maintains a strong, healthy body. When it does the opposite of any of these, exercise may actually be a detriment, severely interfering with your healing efforts. Indeed, exercise is potentially a great detoxifier, breathing support, and healer of mild anxiety or sadness, but only when it is done in a way that honours the whole self. As helpful as exercise can be in some circumstances, rest—even long periods of it—can be just as or more important. As you progress through GAPS, ask yourself: "At this particular phase in my healing journey, does my body need rest to reach its next level? Or does it need movement?" The answer will vary from day to day, season to season, and year to year. At any given time, it will be different for each person.

Fat Malabsorption

Some people coming to GAPS struggle with fat absorption. Some have even had their gall bladder removed. In the *Intro* section of this Guide, I note that if fat malabsorption is an issue for you, you can start with a small amount (even 5 mL or 1 teaspoon) of fat per meal or per day and increase the amount as you are able. Dr. Campbell-McBride also recommends increasing your body's capacity to digest and assimilate fat by taking ox bile with every meal, using coffee enemas, and incorporating a "GAPS milkshake." Dr. Campbell-McBride's shake is made by whisking together fresh, home-pressed juice from fruits and vegetables, one to two raw eggs (both the yolk and the white), and a large dollop of raw sour cream (or coconut oil, if sour cream has not yet been introduced). Start with 2–3 tablespoons of this shake per day, gradually increasing to two glasses per day with one taken first thing in the morning on an empty stomach and the second taken mid-afternoon on an empty stomach. For more information on the benefits of this shake and on ox bile, coffee enemas, and so on, see Dr. Campbell-McBride's FAQ document.

Heart Health

Regarding any concerns about the use of fats in relation to heart health, please see Dr. Campbell-McBride's book *Put Your Heart in Your Mouth: Natural Treatment for Angina, Arrhythmia, Atherosclerosis, Heart Attack, High Blood Pressure, Peripheral Vascular Disease, and Stroke.*

Heartburn, Reflux, and Indigestion

Many people coming to GAPS have a history of heartburn, reflux, indigestion, or other related irritation. Some people find this symptom worsens in early GAPS or even re-establishes itself after a long period of having been symptom-free. Elevated estrogen levels, food allergies, and bacterial overgrowth have all been suggested as possible underlying causes. In GAPS, we aim to resolve this symptom by increasing stomach acid levels. For many, this can be achieved just by doing the basic program. For those for whom this issue persists, I suggest the following:

1. Chew your food (and even your liquids) thoroughly. This can make all the difference in digestive capacity, often preempting any need for remedies.
2. Upon waking, throughout the day, and 10–15 minutes before each meal take:
   - 15 mL (1 tablespoon) apple cider vinegar in a cup of not-cold water;
   - Juice of fermented vegetables; or
   - Juice of fermented vegetables mixed with a bit of meat stock.

Any of the above will increase your stomach acid levels and aid in achieving reflux-free digestion. Over time, you will be able to reduce the frequency of this practice, ultimately requiring just the basic GAPS protocol.

3. Add ginger tea to your daily program. You can also simmer ginger slices in your soups (remove the slices before eating the soup if you cannot tolerate their fibre).

4. If the issue continues after two weeks of consistently trying each of the previous tips, try betaine HCL with pepsin as detailed in the *Supplementation* section of this Guide.

5. Continue slowly increasing your probiotics.

6. Continue increasing your GAPS oils.

7. See the additional tips offered by Dr. Campbell-McBride in her FAQ document.

8. In some people, a single session of physical manipulation, such as chiropractic or specific body movements, has resolved heartburn or reflux. You may wish to ask around your local community for a health practitioner with experience resolving this symptom.

If your symptoms are unbearable during early healing, take the prescription, medicine, or herb that works for you while continuing the healing process. Over time, your dosage of remedy can likely be decreased until you need none at all.

Histamine Intolerance

Many people come to GAPS with this issue, and the program resolves it. Dr. Campbell-McBride recommends that a person with this issue avoid even the GAPS versions of the following in early healing: alcohol, black tea, canned food, smoked food, beans, lentils, fermented vegetables, mature cheeses, cocoa, nuts, and anything else that aggravates your histamine levels. Eat freshly prepared foods, avoiding leftovers as much as possible. For ferments, rely on GAPS yogurt and GAPS kefir. Be sure to incorporate the Intro diet. As with all symptoms, the time required to heal this issue is different for everyone. As with any intolerance, simply keep testing foods every month or so—introducing tomato, eggplant, or spinach before testing fermented vegetables—until your body demonstrates a capacity to process these.

Hypoglycemia/Low Blood Sugar

A number of people coming to GAPS report symptoms of low blood sugar, and quite a few have been diagnosed with hypoglycemia. Many support list members have found that lifelong blood sugar issues resolved very early in GAPS.

Likewise, pre-GAPS I had significant blood sugar issues and on GAPS, none. GAPS is very helpful for these symptoms. Do the program as outlined, including a savoury GAPS meal rich in protein and fat upon waking, every hour or so throughout the day, and right before bed. Sipping on a replenishing drink throughout the day may also help. During early healing and when sugar cravings are strong, Dr. Campbell-McBride recommends mixing raw butter or virgin coconut oil with a bit of raw honey (just enough to accept the taste) in a jar and carrying it with you. Eat 5–15 mL (1–3 teaspoons) of this mixture every 20 minutes or so (more often if needed) throughout the day. She also suggests carrying a second jar of plain coconut oil and eating that regularly, too (note that coconut oil may trigger die-off). As time passes, you will feel fine for longer and longer stretches. For low blood sugar, fatigue, mood swings, or chronic hunger, many GAPSters have had excellent results with shakes or puddings offering an infusion of fats (and in some cases protein), from whatever sources their personal tolerances allow. Common ingredients include coconut oil, sour cream, or butter for fat; raw eggs or homemade whey, yogurt, or kefir for protein; coconut milk or a small amount of honey or fruit for sweetness; and a pinch of salt. Ultimately, the basic GAPS program with three to six savoury meals and snacks per day is all you will need. Please also see the section *Health Issues: Cravings and Hunger*.

Medication

Medication is a challenging topic. On the one hand, medication can relieve symptoms enough that one can actually take on a program such as GAPS. On the other hand, medications themselves trigger concerns about toxins. In addition, Dr. Campbell-McBride does not recommend taking any medication long term. The decision as to whether or not to take medication while healing the body through GAPS needs to be made by you in consultation with your health care practitioner. I will share a few thoughts here, though.

As is obvious through my own story presented at the opening of this book, I benefited greatly from the temporary use of (psychiatric) medication. In my opinion, although there are risks with some medications, just as there are with any other changes to one's lifestyle, there is no need to take an absolute stance for or against the use of medication. Some people are in severe physical or mental distress and have few options for immediate relief or support. Medications may provide them with enough resources (e.g., physical strength or cognitive clarity) to take on the program. Pre-GAPS, it was in starting a one-year course of Paxil® that I became able to think clearly enough to shop and cook, as well as to participate in enough therapy to inspire a long-term commitment to my health. Medications required to preserve life or limb should be continued for as long as needed, including while on GAPS. These include medications that halt excessive bleeding or incapacitating pain, for example, but also those that prevent other forms of harm to self or others, such as suicide, self-injury, and aggression.

Whether the medication is to treat psychosis, hypothyroidism, Crohn's disease, an acute infection, or anxiety, your healing will continue to progress. As it does so, you may find yourself becoming increasingly sensitive to the medication. That is, you may begin noticing side effects not previously felt. When this is the case, discuss matters with your health care practitioner who may adjust your dose or type of medication.

Through GAPS, many people do see their need for medication greatly reduced or eliminated over time. When healing seems to be taking a firm hold, a conversation with your health care practitioner may result in the slow reduction of medication. By reducing it in small increments, you will have an opportunity to assess the effects of the reduced amount. In any case, one should not suddenly stop any medications because doing so can trigger other symptoms, including life-threatening ones. Rather, allow GAPS time to do its work, and take any medication-related steps gently and cautiously in consultation with your health care practitioner. Your healing journey can and should be relatively comfortable as well as safe. Finally, if the medication in question is an antibiotic, be sure to continue taking probiotics (at a different time of the day) during its course.

Severe Intestinal Issues

Folks coming to GAPS with issues such as chronic diarrhea, Crohn's disease, or ulcerative colitis have some additional considerations. One key will be to regard your body as a sensitive one. Accordingly, be sure to start your probiotic dose, for example, according to the directions given within this Guide for a "very ill or very sensitive adult" and approach fibrous and advanced foods with extra caution, testing only one at a time and starting with a very small amount of each. The following points should also be considered.

Transitioning/Intro: The severity of your symptoms may be such that you are best served by skipping the slow transition presented in this Guide and starting Intro as soon as you have your supplies. The relief experienced in early Intro—with its earliest stages offering freedom from the most aggravating foods, a rapid healing, and a gradual introduction of the more complex foods—may well outweigh the discomfort otherwise triggered in jumping right in. (If taking this approach, still be sure to read the information in this entire Guide before beginning. Information and tips within each section will be important to your overall journey.)

Eggs: These trigger diarrhea in a number of people. Intro's earliest forms (e.g., yolks in soup or soft-boiled) may be fine, but scrambled eggs trigger looser stools in many people. If this is true for you, continue with the forms your body accepts and omit the forms that cause you difficulty. Retest the problematic forms after some additional weeks of healing.

Fruit: Although ripe bananas may be fine, the fibre in other raw fruits may aggravate the intestines.

Lentils, beans, and split peas: After you have been free of diarrhea for at least three months, dried legumes can be tested, but these should be fermented. Proper preparation may make all the difference (see *Recipes: Ferments–Beans*).

Juices: These may be a problem early on, especially citrus ones (e.g., orange juice). Coconut water is also reported to trigger diarrhea in some people.

Nuts and nut flours: Nuts and nut flours often trigger looser stools. As with anyone doing GAPS, nuts in any form should be severely limited in quantity. Soaking and/or fermenting them may make all the difference to tolerance (see *Recipes: More Essentials–Nuts and Seeds*).

Vegetables: As many folks with severe intestinal issues can attest, it is fine to avoid vegetables for the first several weeks, and it may be very helpful to do so. When you are ready to test vegetables, start with soft, well-cooked, peeled, de-seeded ones. For example, carrots and peeled, de-seeded zucchini are generally safe to start with. (Tip: A large zucchini will offer a much higher flesh-to-seed ratio than a smaller one will.) Cruciferous vegetables may be especially challenging (e.g., bok choy, broccoli, Brussels sprouts, cabbage, cauliflower, kale, and watercress). Introduce these with caution. Start with none, and then include small amounts of the less-fibrous parts, such as florets versus stalks, all well-cooked and eaten with broth. Over time, you will be able to include increased quantities of vegetables, and more of any vegetable's fibrous sections. Ferments can initially be limited to water- or coconut-based ones, cabbage rejuvelac, ones made from less-fibrous vegetables (e.g., carrots), and dairy forms (e.g., kefir).

Small Intestine Bacterial Overgrowth (SIBO)

Whether diagnosed with SIBO or not, many people coming to GAPS have a chronic bacterial infection of the small intestine. The GAPS program will resolve it. Dr. Allison Siebecker (www.siboinfo.com) is available for consultation specific to this issue.

Weight

See *Progressing Further: Weight adjustments.*

CHAPTER 13

FOOD ISSUES

Commonly Relied-Upon Foods

When we rely upon any one food more than another, we can run into a number of issues. We may inadvertently begin narrowing our food range, perpetuating cravings for sweet foods, gravitating toward foods more difficult to digest, and so on. These habits commonly apply to fruit, nuts, and dairy, but may apply to any food. It is also quite common to have a strong dependence on a food that we are reactive to, which only perpetuates the sensitivity and the craving for it.

In this section of the Guide, I discuss reliance on any food we either (1) use in excess, or (2) refuse to rotate out, even in support of deeper healing. I use dairy as an example, but the concepts apply equally to any other food.

Dairy

For people who tolerate it, GAPS recommends the inclusion of home-fermented or otherwise lactose-free dairy. These products (e.g., yogurt or kefir fermented at least 24 hours, certain cheeses, ghee, or butter) provide vital vitamins and minerals, satiate the body, transport copious friendly bacteria and yeasts, and provide variety in flavour, texture, and meal options. Initially, even these excellent dairy options may need to be avoided. Small amounts of residual lactose or the presence of casein (a milk protein) may cause problems for some people. A compromised gut may require some healing before these can be reintroduced. (Dr. Campbell-McBride also recommends that people with breast cysts avoid dairy and other sources of xenoestrogens until the cysts have resolved.)

Some people do well introducing home-fermented whey, sour cream, yogurt, and/or kefir from very early on. Others do not. For one person, even GAPS dairy may trigger constipation, diarrhea, eczema, or other symptoms; for another, home-fermented dairy may actually resolve these issues. Just like every other GAPS food, even home-fermented dairy will need to be tested by each individual.

It is not possible to know in advance who will benefit most from keeping dairy out of their program and who will benefit most by adding it into their program. The safest approach for most people seems to be as follows: Start Intro without dairy, keep it out for at least two weeks, and then introduce it according to the guidelines at the end of this section (for those skipping Intro, a different schedule of dairy introduction is offered in Dr. Campbell-McBride's book *Gut and Psychology Syndrome*).

People with a known or suspected sensitivity to dairy might choose the conservative approach of keeping all dairy out for six weeks before testing it.

Keeping dairy out for two (or six) weeks, starting from Day 1 of Intro, offers many potential benefits:

- **A full digestive rest from dairy's sugar (lactose) and its more challenging protein (casein)**. Even raw or fermented dairy is hard for some people to digest. I like to see a person's healing program open with the lightest, easiest, gentlest, fastest, most effective approach to healing. I believe that for most people (although not necessarily all), excluding dairy temporarily is one aspect of this. A dairy-free period can make all the difference in one's healing, and can allow ghee, butter, and fermented dairy to be introduced earlier than it otherwise might.

- **Identification of intolerance**. The methodical elimination and subsequent reintroduction of a substance can help identify a strong intolerance.

- **Motivation to rely on marrow, tissues, broth, eggs, vegetable ferments, fats from the insides of animals, etc.** These are very healing foods, yet many bodies in a compromised state veer away from them and toward old standbys. Giving ourselves the option to rely on our previous approaches, such as weekly dairy, can keep us in a perpetual state of compromised health.

- **A movement toward creativity**. In Canada, a dairy advertisement relying on reverse psychology screeches, "Can't get your [adult] kids to leave home?! Stop cooking with cheese!" The implication is that cheese makes everything taste great, and that nothing without it can taste good. Pre-GAPS, I lived that philosophy: cheese on toast, cheese on broccoli, cheese as an entire meal, cheese to top an already protein-rich lentil loaf...It wasn't until I gave up dairy and was forced to find other sources of "delish" that I finally came to appreciate the flavour of dairy-free dishes, and also became able to invent them ad hoc. That is, I learned how to bring other ingredients together for equally satisfying results. By excluding dairy for a period of time, I created a new habit of relying on eggs, meats, vegetables, vegetable ferments, and non-dairy sources of fat. This has served me very well, including long after I reintroduced dairy into our diets. Every time I remove dairy from our diet, my son also regains a stronger interest in a wider range of foods.

All of these points apply equally to any other GAPS foods that we tend to rely on (e.g., nuts, nut flours, and fruits) over marrow, tissues, meats, eggs, fats from the inside of an animal, ferments, and broths. With rare exception, I prefer to see 4-6 weeks of Intro free of our commonly craved foods, frequently used ingredients, and so on. My son and I did not use dairy for our first weeks of GAPS, and then we used just ghee for about 6 months. We then introduced yogurt, then kefir, then cheese. Because it benefits us to do so, we still regularly cycle dairy, nuts, and/or fruit out of our personal programs for 1-6 weeks at a time.

So, how long is it really necessary to exclude dairy or any other food? Again, every person is different, and every decision you make about your program is your own. If your intuition, body, or health practitioner says to include dairy or another food earlier in your program and this works for you, I celebrate this! Regardless of when you opt to include dairy, following are some guidelines.

Which milk? If the only milk available to you is commercial, pasteurized cow's milk, feel free to use that to make your yogurt, kefir, and so on. If properly fermented, even commercial milk will be abundant in health-giving bacteria and tolerated by most people. Of course, non-organic, factory-processed cow's milk will carry some degree of toxins, such as antibiotics, and a form of casein more difficult to digest by some people than that present in the milk of some other animals. People who are sensitive to "regular" milk or those who can afford a cleaner version might consider milk from another animal (e.g., goat or camel), and/or raw milk, and/or milk free of pesticides and antibiotics (i.e., organic). These tend to be more easily digested and/or will bring fewer toxins into your body. The GAPS community views raw milk as a very healthy post-GAPS food, but for the healing belly it is included only in the same forms as any other milk (i.e., as ghee, butter, or a fermented product). Milk that is soured, as opposed to fermented, is not used in GAPS.

When? If one is doing the Intro progression, healing is quicker, thus dairy can be tested quite early on. Most people doing Intro will tolerate homemade ghee and/or home-fermented whey by late Stage 3. The point in Intro when whey is first introduced (in a recipe for fermented fish) is usually 2 or more weeks into Intro. Once you have been free of dairy for at least 2 weeks, try 5 mL (1 teaspoon) of home-fermented whey, preferably as part of the *Fermented Fish* recipe (it does not have to be measured; a bite of the fish will suffice), but otherwise in any other form, including directly off a spoon. Slowly and methodically, work up from there and then on to other GAPS-friendly dairy products at your own pace, as outlined at the end of this section.

If skipping Intro, your body will require much more time to heal. In this case, do not use any dairy except ghee for 6 weeks. After 6 weeks, test butter. After an additional 6–12 weeks with just ghee and butter, test 5 mL (1 teaspoon) of GAPS yogurt or sour cream. Gradually increase the amount. When at least 80 mL (⅓ cup) is tolerated, test 5 mL (1 teaspoon) of kefir. When at least 80 mL (⅓ cup) of kefir is tolerated, test a mouthful of cheddar cheese. When all of these have been successfully introduced, try other GAPS cheeses.

Whey, Yogurt, or Kefir? All home-fermented options are excellent. Their proteins are predigested or denatured, allowing them to be used relatively early in healing even by many people with the most troubled bellies. Home-fermented whey contains the bacterial properties of yogurt, but without yogurt's potentially aggravating protein casein (which can be problematic for some bellies early in healing, even when denatured). Yogurt, on the other hand, contains healthy bacteria plus the bonus of excellent fats, as well as flavour and texture that lends itself well to many recipes. Kefir includes all of these benefits plus healthy yeasts that can help balance an overgrowth of *Candida,* for example. Because yogurt generally produces a milder response in the body, Dr. Campbell-McBride suggests people incorporate yogurt before kefir.

To Start: Assuming you are doing Intro, after at least 2-6 weeks without dairy a very sensitive person might start with 5 mL (1 teaspoon) or less of whey per day and work up slowly, perhaps doubling the dose every 3-7 days, as your sensitivity or degree of die-off allows. Once 80 mL (⅓ cup) of whey is tolerated, add 5 mL (1 teaspoon) or less of yogurt or home-fermented sour cream per day to your program, and work slowly up. Once at least 80 mL (⅓ cup) of yogurt or sour cream is tolerated, begin adding 5 mL (1 teaspoon) or less of kefir per day to that. Slowly increase the amount of kefir. When you can tolerate 250 mL (1 cup) of kefir, enjoy this regularly, as well as yogurt and sour cream if desired. Allow your body to determine how little or how much yogurt, kefir, or other dairy to consume in any given day or week. Any time after this process and all of Intro has been completed, test butter, and then GAPS cheese.

Food Sensitivities/Allergies

"I've never noticed any reaction to dairy/rice/fruit. Do I really have to eliminate this?" • *"I'm reactive to almost every food. How will I do the program?"* • *"Why after starting GAPS do I react to foods I didn't react to pre-GAPS?"* • *"I'm allergic to phenols—wouldn't doing a low-phenol version of GAPS be too restricted?"*

> **! IMPORTANT**
>
> When an allergic reaction (even a non-anaphylactic one) can be life-threatening, consult with your health practitioner and test foods only under her advice and supervision.

Many allergies, sensitivities, and intolerances seem to be linked to a compromised gut. GAPS aims to resolve this. Consequently, we see most sensitivities resolve, including immunoglobulin E (IgE) allergies and responses to environmental elements such as pollen. But this process takes time (this is why the program is at least 18–24 months long).

Do not underestimate the power of GAPS to heal the gut lining! Through the program, the gut will become able to properly process healthy foods previously not tolerated. As the physical holes in the gut wall heal, and the microvilli heal and substantial bacterial levels are established, foods can be digested without a reaction. Many people who have started or completed the GAPS program are now eating a variety of foods they had not been able to consume for years: dairy, nuts, and eggs are common examples. They approached the program with care and attention and have found fabulous results! A mother on one of our e-mail support lists reports that her child has eosinophilic esophagitis—the child's esophagus would close whenever she ingested dairy. Dr. Campbell-McBride suggested this mother introduce whey by dipping the tip of a knife into the whey, mixing the whey with broth, and then serving it. The child was able to ingest this without reaction (when tried previously, the same amount without broth had caused the throat to close).

In the meantime, the inability to eat specific foods need not be a problem. Many people do many weeks or months of GAPS without dairy, eggs, nuts, certain meats, whole vegetables, fermented vegetables, or any other GAPS food (including the broth in a few cases). As noted in the *Intro* section of this Guide, a diet which includes marrow, soft tissues, eggs or any meats (including fish), fats, vegetables (juiced or otherwise), and a source of probiotics is sufficient. (Some people actually experience optimal health when excluding all carbohydrates, even juiced vegetables.) For those whose bodies demand a simpler diet, but who still crave variety, consider options such as milks made from nuts, kefir made from coconut water, ice cream made from frozen bananas, breads made from mashed navy beans, and flours made from pecans or coconuts. There are GAPS recipes and/or menu plans available for dairy-free GAPS, egg-free GAPS, and more. For detailed recipes, menus, or video or pictorial instructions, please do an Internet search for the item of your choice. Including "GAPS" in your search (e.g., "GAPS coffee cake") will often bring up wonderful GAPS-specific recipes by bloggers around the world. However, do not limit yourself to GAPS-specific sources. Many recipes from other sources are inherently GAPS-friendly or are easily modified for the program.

Food reactions are very individual. There is no one food that is a perfect fit for everyone all the time. Also, a food you reacted to in the past might be well tolerated when combined with broth or fermented foods, or when some digestive healing has been established. Conversely, a food that was not identified as a problem in the past may suddenly show an ugly side. For example, as a vegetarian, beans were a staple of my diet for over 20 years. I suffered long-term "low-grade" health issues, but from day to day I showed no obvious reaction to legumes, pulses, or beans. Upon starting my healing journey, I removed all of these for several months before reintroducing white beans. They had never seemed problematic before, so I didn't anticipate any trouble. I guess that's why I ate two big bowlfuls of my home-baked bean casserole! Oops! I had gas like I had never known before. (I might have avoided this reaction by following my own advice to introduce items in broth and to start with a small amount!)

I now believe I had been reacting to legumes, beans, and/or pulses throughout my entire life, but that by eating them so regularly, my body had become unable to kick up enough fuss for me to notice. Indeed, it is common for people, pre-GAPS, to react to foods without realizing it. Regular consumption of our trigger foods causes our bodies to display low-grade issues (e.g., headache, joint pain, sadness, or fatigue). When we give the body a sufficient break from trigger foods and then reintroduce them, we often experience an intense, obvious, acute reaction (e.g., migraine, rashes, or depression). One has actually been reacting all along, but with chronic ingestion, the body is so pummeled it can't even get up the gumption to scream anymore! Even those who had not noticed a reaction to a given food previously, including a GAPS food during their GAPS program, have found great gains in temporarily eliminating it from their diet.

Resolving Food Sensitivities

Step 1: Support Digestion

A primary approach to eliminating reactions is to simply support digestion. Tips for doing so are detailed throughout this Guide, but I will review them briefly here. Throughout the day, and at least 15 minutes before each meal, sip from a glass of room temperature water with 15 mL (1 tablespoon) of apple cider vinegar added to it. Include broth and a fermented food or drink with each meal. Try a troublesome food mixed with broth. Drink any other fluids at least 30 minutes before or 2½ hours after meals. While eating, chew your food very thoroughly. At least once daily, and preferably two to three times, clear your body's digestive tract through a bowel movement. At any point in the day, gently and kindly massage your abdomen. For at least 30 minutes over the course of a day, walk gently in the fresh air or do gentle stretches. Get lots of rest. As much as possible, avoid stress. If you are still struggling after implementing all these approaches, try betaine HCL with pepsin in your program. It's amazing how many "food intolerances" are resolved quickly and inexpensively by incorporating one or more of these approaches!

Step 2: Identify Allergenic vs. Detoxifying Foods

Any group of foods may trigger a reaction in an individual. For you, the problematic group may be nightshades (e.g., eggplant, peppers, and tomatoes), crucifers (e.g., broccoli, cauliflower, Brussels sprouts, kale, and cabbage), foods rich in sulphur (e.g., cabbage, broccoli, and onions), citrus fruits, or foods high in oxalates, phenols, or salicylates. Each of these groups of foods has strong nutritional and/or detoxification properties. Thus, a reaction to them may indicate detoxification, which is desirable. As with all GAPS foods, they should be included if possible (they will not be a problem for most people, or an initial reaction will be resolved through the normal GAPS progression). However, some people are very sensitive to the effects of specific foods and experience significant discomfort upon ingesting them. If you suspect that your body reacts strongly to a detoxifying food or element, such as salicylates or oxalates (do an Internet search for foods containing high amounts of the element under suspicion), remove the element for two to six weeks, and then retest it using the "low and slow method" just as one would with any other powerful food, such as yogurt, coconut oil, or a yeast killer. If you try several times to reintroduce a food and it continues to trigger discomfort, feel free to remove it for some weeks or months (or even years). Just as with GAPS, there are wonderful websites and e-mail lists to support people who need to exclude any given element from their diet, including in combination with GAPS.

Again, I do not recommend restricting the diet too deeply at the beginning. Rather, I recommend that you initially do the program as laid out, excluding only those foods that you know you cannot tolerate. If after a few months you sense that some tweaking is necessary, you can test any food or food group. As always, the only way to know if a period of elimination is necessary is by trial. Many people find that by severely reducing the presence of a given element (e.g., salicylates) in their diet for just two to six weeks, the element can be reintroduced in limited, and then increasing, amounts. When reintroducing these elements, allow for some degree of healing effect. Only if our bodies are truly overwhelmed should we consider limiting them further.

WHEN DOES A REACTION INDICATE INTOLERANCE VERSUS DIE-OFF OR A HEALING CRISIS?

Often, there is no way to know. Eczema, constipation, and diarrhea are common to both intolerance and die-off, and a healing crisis can be triggered simply by adding an especially powerful food to our program. When we know that a food is probiotic (e.g., kefir), antifungal (e.g., coconut oil), or detoxifying (e.g., grapefruit), we can reasonably conclude that any "reactions" indicate die-off or healing crisis. In these cases, we can reduce to a lower amount, if that feels necessary. Otherwise, gently push through the symptoms, implementing lots of die-off relief strategies in the meantime. If you react to a food that is not known to be especially probiotic, antifungal, or detoxifying, it is reasonable to view the reaction as an indication that the food is not currently tolerated. In these cases, you can follow the steps offered subsequently for the "low and slow method" and "elimination and reintroduction." As we proceed through the program, we come to know our own bodies. After some weeks or months, we gain a sense of which symptoms indicate intolerance and which indicate die-off. Unfortunately, there is no shortcut to obtaining this knowledge. Proceeding very slowly can help. Regardless of the cause, the die-off relief approaches can help very much during an increase in symptoms (see *Relief from Transitional Discomfort*).

Step 3: Low and Slow Method

To distinguish a true allergy from a healing crisis, to keep reactions manageable, or to increase your body's capacity for a strongly healing element, follow the "low and slow" method of introducing new items.

Day 1: Introduce 5 mL (1 teaspoon) or less.

Day 2: Leave the new food out.

Day 3: If no reaction to date, introduce 15 mL (3 teaspoons).

Day 4: Leave the new food out.

Day 5: If still no reaction, use the new food freely (sensitive people may wish to continue increasing slowly).

If introducing even 5 mL (1 teaspoon) on its own triggers a reaction, leave the food out for another month, then try this process again, this time including the food within a larger meal.

Step 4: Test for Sensitivities

If the previous steps do not resolve a reaction to a given food, test for sensitivities using one of the methods presented in the *Testing for Food Sensitivities* section. In the meantime, if it is chicken eggs you are reacting to, for example, try eggs from ducks or geese. If beef is problematic, try lamb, buffalo, or salmon instead. If you react to even pastured meat, try wild meats.

Step 5: Assess Carbohydrate Sensitivity

An additional issue common to GAPSters is that of carbohydrate sensitivity. As discussed earlier, GAPS does not aim to limit the amount of carbohydrates one ingests. Rather, it proposes eating mostly (though not entirely) a specific type of carbohydrate (monosaccharides) versus another (polysaccharides). Some people are especially sensitive to carbohydrate counts, regardless of the type or source. This is often true for people whose diets were heavy in carbohydrates pre-GAPS, for example.

People sensitive to carbohydrates may react quite obviously to the sugars in carrots, orange squash (e.g., butternut), fruit, honey, and nuts. The early stages of Intro are very helpful for addressing this. If you react to carbohydrates—whether immediately with mood swings, after an hour or so with fatigue, or over weeks or months with a slow, insidious gain of excess weight—you may need to address this sensitivity head on. One way is to simply rely on marrow, soft tissues, meats, eggs, broths, fats, ferments, and non-orange vegetables for several weeks or months. (Other vegetables also have carbohydrates, but the count is lower; in some vegetables, the fibre count brings the carbohydrate count effectively to nil.) After preparing for the program and enjoying Full GAPS for a time, start with Intro's Stage 1 but initially include only non-sweet items in the earliest stages of your progression. If you are including vegetables, and eating freely, you will still be getting carbohydrates. After a few days of this, add a small amount of a carbohydrate-rich, stage-friendly food (e.g., butternut squash or carrots) and observe your body's response. A response of relaxation and grounded energy, with no adverse symptoms, is a sign that your body can tolerate that amount of carbohydrate, and possibly more.

If increasing your carbohydrate count causes symptoms such as mood swings, inexplicable fatigue, or unwanted weight gain, you can try to pinpoint your current tolerance. For some people, the following approach may be helpful: Start or restart with Intro's Stage 1, but use only animal products. After 2 or 3 days, start incorporating 10 grams of carbohydrates (from vegetables) into your program every day for one week. If symptoms resurface, return to a diet of just animal products; continue with just animal products for several weeks before testing 10 grams again. After each week that you are symptom-free on a given level of carbohydrates, you might increase your carbohydrate count by another 10 grams per day, such that you will be ingesting approximately 20 grams per day for a week, then 30 grams per day for a week, and so on.

While many adults experience maximum health on 80–150 grams of carbohydrates per day, some function optimally on 150-400 grams or more of GAPS carbohydrates per day, while still others can tolerate only zero or 10 grams per day for a time. Carbohydrate tolerance can vary with age, activity level, and a host of other variables. Also, many people are sensitive to carbohydrates just at the beginning of healing. It is important to realize that this will resolve over some months. When a sensitivity to carbohydrates has healed, continued restriction of healthy carbohydrates may become a problem, triggering crankiness and fatigue at the very least. Listen to your body. It will ask for fewer or more GAPS carbohydrates at any given point, and it is important to honour such requests.

Step 6: Neutralization or Desensitization

When faster or additional support with food intolerances, sensitivities, or allergies is required, neutralization may be effective. Many GAPSters have reported excellent results with approaches such as homeopathy, Nambudripad's Allergy Elimination Techniques (NAET), and others. However, do not underestimate the power of proper digestive practices (e.g., chewing), GAPS itself, Intro, and the "low and slow method" of reintroduction in resolving intolerances. Many sensitivities are successfully addressed through the basic GAPS program, eliminating the need for additional effort or expense.

Testing for Food Sensitivities

> **REMEMBER**
>
> When a food or item has previously triggered a serious reaction, test it only under the guidance and supervision of a health practitioner.

If food sensitivities are present, you may have to introduce some foods later than the program suggests. If you suspect a sensitivity to a particular food, test it before introducing it. There are a number of methods by which you can do this.

Elimination and Reintroduction: This is my preferred form of test for most people. Select a food (e.g., plum), food group (e.g., fruit), or food element (e.g., salicylates). A group can be anything you decide: fibrous, high oxalate, nightshade, sweet, and so on. Do an Internet search to find a complete list of foods falling within a given category. Ensure no amount of this food, group, or element is ingested for an entire two weeks. Watch for any changes in mood, behaviour, skin, and so on. After two or more weeks, reintroduce the food, group, or element. Use quite a bit of it every day for a few days. Over the subsequent week, watch for changes in mood, behaviour, skin, and so on. If reintroduction of the food or element triggers an obvious reaction, leave it out for another month, then try the food, group, or element again, this time using the "low and slow method" of food reintroduction.

If your test involved a group of foods and there was a reaction, at some point test individual "members" of that group to see whether it is a specific food or the entire category of food that is triggering it.

Testing Intro Foods: Intro is essentially a form of "elimination and reintroduction" for many foods at once. Because it starts with just a handful of foods—and less commonly allergenic ones at that—the Intro progression is a great way to test for sensitivities. The catch? Some people have an intolerance to the foods they included even on Stages 1 and 2! If you plan to do Intro, but suspect that one or more Intro foods may be problematic for you, you can do one of two things:

1. Before starting Intro, do "elimination and reintroduction" with suspected foods. If any trigger a reaction, leave them out for the first 2 weeks of Intro.

2. Alternatively, proceed through Intro as presented, avoiding any foods you suspect will trigger major problems. When your range of food has built up to a wide variety, eventually rotate out the earliest foods you included. That is, if you chose to include beef meat and beef broth from Stage 1 and subsequently come to suspect beef as being problematic for you, test it whenever you have successfully introduced enough other foods that you need not rely on beef.

Muscle Testing: Some members of the GAPS community have found muscle testing to be very helpful. Although approaches to this simple and free activity vary, essentially one observes the loss or gain of the body's vigour when in contact with a given element. (Without having known a thing about muscle testing, I pinpointed my prenatal vitamin as the source of my intense nausea simply by noticing my body's very strong reaction to the bottle as I walked past and glanced at it! My family physician subsequently confirmed that the supplement's iron content was the trigger for my persistent and extreme vomiting.) Look online or in books for descriptions or videos of how to do muscle testing, or ask a natural health practitioner to teach you.

Skin Test: Skin tests can be administered by a professional or done at home but, like blood tests, they can display inconsistent results. Thus, I am not a big fan of them. Dr. Campbell-McBride offers one approach that may show the presence of a strong allergy in some cases: Before bed, take a drop of the food (mash and mix with a bit of water if the food is solid) and place it on the inside of a wrist. Let the drop dry on the skin, then go to sleep. In the morning, check the spot. If there is an "angry red" reaction, avoid that food for a few weeks (then retest). Note that a lack of reaction is not definitive. That is, if there is no reaction, it is unknown whether or not your body tolerates the food. In this case, you might next test the food using the "low and slow method."

In GAPS, it is common to find most food intolerances resolved after a period of healing. In most cases, there is no reason to leave a food, group, or element out of one's diet permanently. Do not underestimate the body's capacity to heal! A food you could not tolerate in Week 1, 7, or 12 may become accepted—and very nourishing—to the body after just a few more weeks of healing. This is one of the main purposes of GAPS. Be sure to retest foods, incorporating over time as many of GAPS' nutrient-dense foods as possible.

CHAPTER 14
RECIPES: SOUPS FOR INTRO

In this section I present some ideas for basic soups. First, here are some tips that apply to any GAPS soups, including those for the earliest stages of Intro.

- Omit any ingredient from any of the following soup recipes (e.g., onions or apple cider vinegar) that you cannot tolerate yet. Apple cider vinegar helps to draw minerals from the soup bones, but it is not essential for meat broths.

- Any non-fibrous GAPS vegetable that you tolerate is fine to use from the very beginning. Any one or more of celery, cabbage, peas, onions, kale, etc., may be too fibrous for some initially; large pieces of these can be included in the simmer to add flavour and then strained out before serving.

- Measured raw, I use up to 3.5 litres (15 cups) of vegetables per 0.5 kg (1 lb) of meat. People with aggravated intestinal tracts will use smaller amounts of vegetables, or none at all. To create variety in flavours, I often concentrate just one or two main veggies (beyond the onion and garlic) into any soup.

- I typically cook just one soup per day, saving some from each batch for subsequent days. Therefore, after three days on Intro, I have three different soups to choose from at any point during that day.

- Ginger is an excellent digestive aid, but ginger root is fibrous and may be too challenging for some people. As with all ingredients in these recipes, feel free to leave it out. Alternatively, include large, coarsely sliced pieces of ginger in the simmer to provide additional flavour and digestive support, and then remove the pieces before serving (or work around them in your soup bowl).

- Add freshly crushed peppercorns to a soup from the start of its simmer. This will aid digestion. At the beginning of most soup recipes, I direct you to add these at the beginning. Coarsely crushed peppercorns may be too difficult for a child to manage, in which case you can crush them finely before adding them to the soup pot, remove them from the soup after cooking, or blend the entire batch of soup with an immersion blender. At the end of each recipe, I direct you to add additional, finely ground pepper to the soup pot (or to each serving bowl), as your taste dictates.

- In many recipes, I rely on the fat provided by the animal parts, such as chicken thighs or meaty lamb bones. In recipes relying on a less fatty meat, such as sole fillets, I direct you to add fat directly. It is good practice to add additional fat to any soup, whether the soup uses leaner animal cuts or fattier ones.

- In early stages, supplementary fat can be duck fat, tallow, the solids from on top of a broth, and so on. In later stages or Full GAPS, it can also be ghee, butter, leftover bacon grease, or coconut oil.

- I include garlic from the beginning of most soup recipes. This is to allow the flavour to infuse the soup. Whether or not you do this, Dr. Campbell-McBride recommends that those who tolerate garlic add a minced clove of it at the end of the soup's simmer, bring the soup back up to a boil, and then immediately shut the heat off. If doing this, for each soup recipe have available one more clove of garlic than the recipe calls for. Some chefs recommend avoiding even a brief boil so as to maintain the integrity of gelatin and other key elements of broth. Which approach to use is up to you.

- In a pinch, if you are using boneless meat (as opposed to meat on bones and joints) and plain water (as opposed to broth) add a small piece of bone to any soup from any animal you know you tolerate.

- It is fine to use a crockpot or slow-cooker (but not a pressure cooker) for any GAPS meal. The instructions in this Guide assume you are using a basic pot.

- Many people, especially children, prefer their soups, stews, or sauces blended. A "stick," "immersion," or "wand" blender allows you to blend right inside the pot with a simple clean up.

- Our appetites can vary tremendously, so a soup made with a whole chicken plus 3.5 litres (15 cups) of vegetables may last my son and me 24 hours (if experiencing a healing phase's intense hunger and eating only soup in a day) or many meals over several days. If I make a soup in the morning, we might enjoy it for breakfast, fill insulated food containers with it for lunch, and finish it at supper or at any meal the next day. Alternatively, we will refrigerate or freeze some of it for later.

- The following can be refrigerated for up to 1 week. Except for the "noodles" or "rice", they will also keep well in the freezer for up to 3 months.

Stage 1 Soups

Dried herbs are not added until late Stage 2 of Intro, onions are not sautéed until late Stage 3, and meat is not browned until Stage 4. For Stages 1–3, the following process can be used with any meat, including fish, and any GAPS vegetable(s). Although I strongly prefer the soup options available from Stage 4 onward (those which allow the caramelizing of onions, the sautéing of celery, the addition of herbs, and the browning of meat), I present below some early Intro combinations I use. During the soup-intensive stages of the program I might have two mini-meals of the Basic Soup, two of Chicken "Noodle" soup, and two of Cod Mushroom Soup, Beef "Rice" Soup, or whatever other combination I come up with. Thus, even though I'm having soup, soup, and more soup, my need for variety is still satisfied.

Stage 1: 30-Minute Soups

If you have some broth already made (see *Recipes: More Essentials*), you can make a soup this way: To the broth, add any uncooked meat and any tolerated (and generally non-fibrous) GAPS vegetables. Simmer for 30 minutes, regularly skimming off any foam from the top. Dr. Campbell-McBride recommends that you then add 15 mL (1 tablespoon) of minced garlic, bring the soup just to a boil, and shut it off. Before serving, you can also add tissues and meat previously drawn from the bones and joints when you made the broth.

Butternut Squash (Ginger) Soup

Ingredients (makes 1 litre/1 quart):

1	medium butternut squash, peeled and coarsely chopped
500–750 mL (2–3 cups)	chicken broth
2	garlic cloves, minced
15 mL (1 tbsp)	crushed peppercorns
1	yellow onion, chopped
1-2	thumb-sized pieces of ginger, peeled and minced (or coarsely sliced)
60 mL (¼ cup)	fat
2.5 mL (½ tsp)	black pepper, finely ground

For detailed information and variation options, be sure to review the list of notes opening this section before preparing any soup. Put all desired ingredients into an 8-litre (32-cup or 8-quart) pot. Bring to a near boil and then reduce to a simmer for 30 minutes, regularly skimming off any foam from the top. If you wish, use a sieve to remove any large peppercorn pieces from the pot. To the finished soup, add an additional 15 mL (1 tablespoon) of minced garlic. Bring the soup just to a moment's boil, then shut it off and serve. To each bowl, add additional finely ground black pepper and sea salt to each person's taste.

Stage 1: Basic Soup

Because I prefer to make my food as I go, rather than make broth separately in advance, I use the following method to make most of my soups. This means I'm simmering most of my soups for a good two hours before they are initially served.

Ingredients:

0.5 kg (1 lb)[1]	any meat-on-bone or joints, for example, a whole chicken (remove any plastics from inside and out first), chicken drumsticks or backs, lamb on bone, beef on bone, salmon, etc.
2	medium onions, chopped
15 mL (1 tbsp)	apple cider vinegar (to draw nutrients from the bone)
1	garlic clove, minced
1	thumb-sized piece of ginger, minced or sliced
15 mL (1 tbsp)	crushed peppercorns
0.25–3 L (1–12 cups)	any non-fibrous GAPS vegetable parts that are tolerated (e.g., mushrooms, carrots, zucchini, butternut squash, peas, string beans, bell peppers, etc.)
1–5 L (5–20 cups)	water and/or broth (add more liquid for a thinner soup or less for a heartier soup—although not too little because copious liquid is an important aspect in the early Intro soups)

For detailed information and variation options, be sure to review the list of notes opening this section before preparing any soup. Put all ingredients into an 8-litre (32-cup or 8-quart) pot. Bring to a near boil then reduce to a simmer for two to three hours. Regularly skim any foam off the top. If you wish, use a sieve to remove any large peppercorn pieces and small bones from the pot. To the finished soup, add an additional 15 mL (1 tablespoon) of minced garlic. Bring the soup just to a moment's boil, then shut it off and serve. To each bowl, add additional finely ground black pepper and sea salt to each person's taste.

Stage 1 Soup "Noodles"

In early Intro, vegetables are to be well-boiled. Generally, this means they are simmered for 25-30 minutes or more. Vegetables that are cut very thinly may be simmered for a shorter time; use your judgment. Simply ensure early Intro vegetables are very well-cooked and soft for eating. As you progress through the stages, the following vegetable "noodles" can be cooked for shorter and shorter periods, allowing them to retain more of their shape and texture. Eventually, zucchini noodles can be used raw under spaghetti sauce, for example. If you are a big fan of shapes and textures, you might want to invest in a spiralizer or a spiral slicer, a simple hand-crank tool that allows you to turn vegetables into curls or ribbons (e.g., curly fries or spaghetti noodles).

---

[1] This is an approximate amount, but the actual amount of meat used in this recipe is adaptable to your needs. It can range from a drumstick to a whole chicken, for example. Use an amount appropriate for you.

- **Option A—Spaghetti Squash.** Cut the squash in half lengthwise, remove the seeds, and place the squash skin-side-up in a pot of water. Simmer for 30 minutes (in early Intro). Use a fork to pull the "spaghetti" strands from the shell. Set aside.

- **Option B—Zucchini.** Large zucchini offer much more flesh in relation to seed than small ones do. If you have a spiralizer, you can use that to make long, curly noodles of a consistency comparable to spaghetti. Their relative thickness will hold their texture longer than the apple-peeler approach (following) will. If you do not have a spiralizer, use an apple peeler to "peel" zucchini all the way to its core. Leave the noodles as is (the flat, broad segments can be used in lasagne) or cut the noodles vertically and/or horizontally into short straight pieces for Chicken "Noodle" Soup, for example. Set aside.

Chicken "Noodle" Soup

Ingredients:

1	whole chicken (or any pieces of chicken)
1–2 L (4–8 cups)	zucchini or spaghetti squash "noodles," cut as previously described
15 mL (1 tbsp)	apple cider vinegar (to draw nutrients from the bone)
750 mL (3 cups)	onion, chopped
3	garlic cloves, minced
15 mL (1 tbsp)	crushed peppercorns
0.25–3.5 L (1–15 cups)	tolerated vegetables, chopped (e.g., carrots, cauliflower florets, etc.)
variable	water

For detailed information and variation options, be sure to review the list of notes opening this section before preparing any soup. Make and set aside the vegetable "noodles," as presented previously. Remove any plastics from outside and inside of the chicken. Put all ingredients except the "noodles" into an 8-litre (32-cup or 8-quart) pot. The types and amounts of veggies you use are up to you. One version I like includes just celery and carrots, in equal amounts. Bring to a near boil then reduce to a simmer for two hours, regularly skimming any foam off the top. Add your "noodles." Depending on the thickness of your "noodles," simmer another 5–20 minutes. Remove the chicken. Use a sieve to remove any large peppercorn pieces and small bones from the pot (if using chicken pieces). To the finished soup, add an additional 15 mL (1 tablespoon) of minced garlic. Bring the soup just to a moment's boil, then shut it off. From the chicken, cut off some or all of the meat and soft parts and put them back into the soup (blending those in if you prefer). To each bowl, add additional finely ground black pepper and sea salt to each person's taste. Any remaining chicken can be eaten as is, added to another soup, dipped in the reduced broth of another animal, and so on.

Cod Mushroom Soup

Ingredients (makes 1 litre/1 quart):

0.5 kg (1 lb)	cod (or another white fish such as sole), with or without bones, head, fins, and tail
500–750 mL (2–3 cups)	crimini mushrooms
1	onion, chopped
1	garlic clove, minced
15 mL (1 tbsp)	crushed peppercorns
60 mL (¼ cup)	fat
15 mL (1 tbsp)	apple cider vinegar (to draw nutrients from any bone, if used)
2.5 mL (½ tsp)	black pepper, finely ground
500–750 mL (2–3 cups)	water or meat broth (from any animal)

For detailed information and variation options, be sure to review the list of notes opening this section before preparing any soup. Put all ingredients except the water/broth into an 8-litre (32-cup or 8-quart) pot. Add just enough of the water/broth to cover the contents. If using plain water (as opposed to broth) and fish flesh without bones, heads, fins, and/or tails, add a small piece of bone or joint from any animal you know you tolerate. Bring to a near boil then simmer for 60 minutes, regularly skimming off any foam from the top. Use a sieve to remove any large peppercorn pieces and small bone pieces from the pot. To the finished soup, add an additional 15 mL (1 tablespoon) of minced garlic. Bring the soup just to a moment's boil, then shut it off and serve. To each bowl, add additional finely ground black pepper and sea salt to each person's taste.

Beef "Rice" Soup

Ingredients:

800 g (1.75 lb)	ground beef or beef pieces
1	piece of bone or joints from any tolerated animal
2	garlic cloves, minced
15 mL (1 tbsp)	crushed peppercorns
2	yellow onions, chopped
1	thumb-sized piece of ginger, minced or sliced
15 mL (1 tbsp)	apple cider vinegar (to draw nutrients from the bone)
0.25–3 L (1–12 cups)	vegetables (especially dark ones, such as broccoli or kale, to highlight the whiteness of the "rice"), chopped
60 mL (¼ cup)	fat
2.5 mL (½ tsp)	black pepper, freshly crushed
500–750 mL (2–3 cups)	water or broth (from any animal); use more if including lots of vegetables
1	cauliflower, grated

For detailed information and variation options, be sure to review the list of notes opening this section before preparing any soup. Put all ingredients except cauliflower and water/broth into an 8-litre (32-cup or 8-quart) pot. Add enough of the water/broth to just cover the contents. If using ground beef, break it up so it cooks through. Bring to a near boil, then reduce to a simmer for two hours. Regularly skim any foam off the top. Use a sieve to remove any large peppercorn pieces and small bone pieces from the pot. Add the grated cauliflower and simmer for another 15 minutes. To the finished soup, add an additional 15 mL (1 tablespoon) of minced garlic. Bring the soup just to a moment's boil, then shut it off and serve. To each bowl, add additional finely ground black pepper and sea salt to each person's taste. (In later stages, the grated cauliflower can be added to the simmering soup as few as three minutes before eating. This will help the "rice" to maintain its texture.)

Tomato Chicken Soup

Ingredients (makes 3 litres/3 quarts):

1 kg (2 lb)	chicken parts (e.g., legs and backs), including bones
60 mL (¼ cup)	fat
2 L (8 cups)	tomatoes
1	onion, chopped
1	garlic clove, minced
15 mL (1 tbsp)	crushed peppercorns
15 mL (1 tbsp)	apple cider vinegar (to draw the nutrients from the bone)
750 mL (3 cups)	water
2.5 mL (½ tsp)	black pepper, finely ground

For detailed information and variation options, be sure to review the list of notes opening this section before preparing any soup. Put all ingredients into an 8-litre (32-cup or 8-quart) pot. Bring to a near boil then reduce to a simmer for two to three hours. Regularly skim any foam off the top. Use a sieve to remove (as much as possible in a tomato soup) any large peppercorn pieces and small bones from the pot. To the finished soup, add an additional 15 mL (1 tablespoon) of minced garlic. Bring the soup just to a moment's boil, then shut it off and serve. To each bowl, add additional finely ground pepper and sea salt to each person's taste.

Stages 2 and 3 Soups and Stews

Prepare the soup (more water) or stew (less water), as presented in the previous section. Incorporate the following options as you progress through the stages:

- From the **middle of Stage 2 onward**, as directed at the "stews and casseroles" point of the Intro progression, feel free to add any **fresh herbs**.
- From **late Stage 2 onward**, as directed at the "fermented fish" point of the Intro progression, feel free to add any **dried herbs and additional spices**.
- From **late Stage 2**, you can also add **ghee** to any recipe, if tolerated.
- From **late Stage 3**, you can begin to **sauté onions, then other vegetables such as garlic, celery, and ginger**.

Each of these will make the soups and stews even more delicious.

Stages 4–6: Soups, Stews, Chili, and Spaghetti Sauce

Meat is not browned until the "grilling" point of Stage 4; until that point continue to use the previous soup instructions, and then move on to the following.

The following process is very similar to that presented for Stage 1. The main differences are that you can now sauté items, such as onions, garlic, ginger, and celery, for ten minutes before adding the rest of the ingredients, and you can brown the meat for about ten minutes. These small changes will deeply enhance the soup's flavour.

For any of these four dishes, I start with the same base and "build" the desired recipe from that foundation.

Soup/Stew/Chili/Spaghetti Sauce Base

Ingredients:

125 mL (½ cup)	fat
2	medium onions, chopped
1	garlic clove, minced
1	thumb-sized piece of ginger, minced
15 mL (1 tbsp)	crushed peppercorns
800 g (1.75 lb)	ground beef or other meat
0.25–3 L (1–12 cups)	any vegetables, chopped
1	piece of bone and/or joints
15 mL (1 tbsp)	apple cider vinegar (to draw nutrients from the bone)
5 mL (1 tsp)	black pepper, finely ground
500 mL (2 cups)	celery, chopped (optional)

For detailed information and variation options, be sure to review the list of notes opening this section before preparing any soup. In an 8-litre (approximately 32-cup or 8-quart) pot, heat the fat over medium-high heat. Add onions, garlic, ginger, and/or celery. Sauté until soft, approximately ten minutes. Add the beef, and allow it to brown (approximately another ten minutes). Add the crushed peppercorns and bone/joints. Add any other chopped vegetables that you wish. For my latest batch of stew, I added: 3 medium carrots, 500 mL (2 cups) of kale, and 750 mL (3 cups) of crimini mushrooms. Most GAPS veggies (e.g., zucchini, broccoli, bell peppers, and so on) will work equally well and in any combination. (My own taste buds prefer to pair beets with dill and to generally reserve butternut squash for desserts.) Measured raw, I use in these recipes up to 3.5 litres (15 cups) of vegetables per pound of meat. People with aggravated intestinal tracts, or anyone else who wishes to, will use smaller amounts of vegetables, if any. Depending on the recipe intended, add liquid and/or spices, as follows:

Beef Stew

To the *Soup/Stew/Chili/Spaghetti Sauce Base* detailed above, add only enough water or broth to prevent the contents from burning. Simmer for one to three hours. To the finished stew, add an additional 15 mL (1 tablespoon) of minced garlic. Bring the stew to a moment's boil, then shut it off and serve. Add additional pepper, salt, and 75–125 mL (⅓–½ cup) of ghee to taste.

Beef Soup

To the *Soup/Stew/Chili/Spaghetti Sauce Base* detailed above, add any amount of liquid. For a hearty soup (my preference), add only enough liquid to reach all but the top 5 cm (2 inches) of the pot's contents. Simmer for one to three hours. To the finished soup, add an additional 15 mL (1 tablespoon) of minced garlic. Bring the soup to a moment's boil, then shut it off and serve. Add additional pepper, salt, and 75–125 mL ($\frac{1}{3}$–$\frac{1}{2}$ cup) of ghee to taste.

Spaghetti Sauce

To the *Soup/Stew/Chili/Spaghetti Sauce Base* detailed above add, to your personal taste, approximately 15 mL (1 tablespoon) dried basil, 15 mL (1 tablespoon) dried oregano, 7.5 mL ($\frac{1}{2}$ tablespoon) dried thyme, and tomatoes, as follows. The tomatoes may be pre-cooked and reduced, or fresh (2.5+ litres or 10+ cups), or in the form of 300 mL ($1\frac{1}{4}$ cups) tomato paste, if tolerated. If using fresh tomatoes, allow their juices to release before deciding whether to add any additional liquid. Add a small amount of water or broth to reach desired consistency. Simmer for one to three hours. To the finished sauce, add an additional 15 mL (1 tablespoon) of minced garlic. Bring the sauce to a moment's boil, then shut it off and serve. Add additional pepper, salt, and 75–125 mL ($\frac{1}{3}$–$\frac{1}{2}$ cup) of ghee to taste. Serve over one of the noodle options offered within this Guide. When tolerated, parmesan or cheddar cheese can be grated on top.

Chili

To the *Soup/Stew/Chili/Spaghetti Sauce Base* detailed above, add tomatoes, as follows. The tomatoes may be pre-cooked and reduced, or fresh (2.5+ litres or 10+ cups), or in the form of 300 mL ($1\frac{1}{4}$ cups) tomato paste, if tolerated. If using fresh tomatoes, allow their juices to release before deciding whether to add any additional liquid. Add a small amount of water or broth to reach desired consistency. Add chili spices to your taste. I use approximately 15 mL (1 tablespoon) of chili powder and 15 mL (1 tablespoon) of dried cumin, although people with sensitivity to fillers in mixed spices may need to mix their own chili spice. Simmer for one to three hours. To the finished chili, add an additional 15 mL (1 tablespoon) of minced garlic. Bring the chili to a moment's boil, then shut it off and serve. Add additional pepper, salt, and 75–125 mL ($\frac{1}{3}$–$\frac{1}{2}$ cup) of ghee to taste.

More Soup Flavours!

To the soup base (fat, onions, garlic, etc.) presented in the previous recipes, add any of the following combinations, as appropriate for the stage you are on:

- **Warming:** chopped butternut squash or carrots, lots of ginger slices, and butter
- **Creamy:** lots of broccoli or lots of cauliflower, very little liquid, and blended smooth
- **Light and refreshing:** chicken broth, spiralized and cut zucchini, green onions, and extra water
- **Warm and spicy:** tomatoes and chili spices
- **Tomato:** chopped celery (included in the initial sauté) and heaps of tomatoes
- **Hearty:** cabbage, dill weed, kale, and beets

If you like, you can add meat (e.g., sole, ground beef, salmon, lamb chunks, buffalo pieces, meatballs, or a chicken thigh) to any of these. To the finished soup, add another clove of minced garlic, another 60 mL (¼ cup) of any fat, some pepper to taste, and a fair amount of salt (add, stir, taste; add, stir, taste).

TIP

For many people, a great way to decide what to add is by smelling both the scent coming up from the simmering pot and the ingredient you are considering adding. Not every combination is going to work out as well as others, but through this method, you will very quickly learn how to "throw a soup together."

On the GAPSguide.com website, you will find many more of my original and favourite combinations, as well as links to recipes by many other GAPS bloggers.

CHAPTER 15
RECIPES: FERMENTS

Ferments are simple, yet they can seem very challenging when we first start making them. Leaving dairy or vegetables out on a warm counter for days before ingesting them goes against everything many of us have ever been taught! As a result, many people fear eating or drinking their own initial ferments. I know I did! I refused to try mine for a full month, and did so only after a relative with an ironclad stomach and lots of experience with homemade sauerkraut tried it first. If you are confused or nervous about your batch, ask someone familiar with homemade ferments (e.g., an older neighbour from Eastern Europe or a local member of The Weston A. Price Foundation) to give her opinion on it. When in doubt, throw it out and try again when you are feeling up for another round of work. Don't worry—after a few tries, and perhaps upon locating an alternative method that works better for you, you will get the hang of it!

Fermented Vegetables
Alternatives

I am a strong believer in the use of vegetable ferments. They offer benefits not necessarily offered by other ferments, such as the building of stomach acids needed for digestion. Thus, I encourage people to include vegetable ferments, if tolerated, as well as all other fermentation options. People with histamine intolerance may need to delay the inclusion of fermented vegetables, and instead initially rely on dairy ferments. Also, if you anticipate that you will be unable to tolerate fibre for some time (such as in the case of a severe intestinal disorder like Crohn's disease), feel free to start your program with cabbage rejuvelac, a simple and fast probiotic drink (do an Internet search for "cabbage rejuvelac recipe"). Starting with rejuvelac can also be helpful if you have a large family and will need many portions of juice before introducing actual vegetables.

Benefits

Fermented vegetables (e.g., sauerkraut and kimchi) are a rich source of probiotics and enzymes. They stimulate the secretion of stomach acid when taken before or during a meal, which can help to reduce or resolve reflux, heartburn, or other manifestations of challenged digestion. Some commercial companies are now offering unpasteurized products that may be comparable in benefits to that which we make at home. In terms of cost, accessibility, quality control, and the ability to make quality food directly for ourselves, it is worthwhile to learn to make this at home, even if we opt to use commercial sources at times.

Introducing

Initially, just add the juice of the fermented vegetables into your meals, starting with 5 mL (1 teaspoon) or less per day. If you do not see any juice in your ferment, firmly press a spoon horizontally into the jar and allow the hidden juice to be drawn into the spoon. Each week, increase your dose by another 5 mL (1 teaspoon) or less. When 15 mL (1 tablespoon) of juice is tolerated, start including a bit of the fermented vegetables, if tolerated, into your daily dose.

General Use

Fermented vegetables can be eaten directly from a spoon, added in small or copious amounts to salads, used as one of multiple dressings over a meat patty, or offered as a side dish. Aim to include at least a few teaspoons of fermented food with each meal.

Recipe Options

Some recipes for fermented vegetables call for a fermentation crock, a weight, a loose lid, or an airtight vessel. Please feel free to use any recipe and approach you wish. However, the following directions are tested and accurate for this particular approach. Please do not "mix-and-match" approaches (e.g., largely following this recipe but then keeping the lid loose). Simply follow all the directions, as presented, for whichever method you choose to follow. While many people have had success with batch after batch using the method presented below, many other methods do exist. Sandor Katz (www.wildfermentation.com), for example, is a wonderful resource for a wide range of methods and recipes.

I have included the fermented vegetable recipe I use most often. It is simple and versatile, and pairs nicely with many types of dishes. On the GAPSguide.com website, I offer two more recipes: a Curried Carrot Kraut and a Dill Kraut, the latter of which pairs well with dishes like cabbage rolls and makes a lovely Sour Cream and Dill Veggie Dip when mixed with goat yogurt.

Garlic-Ginger-Veggie Ferment Recipe (Closed Jar Method)

Ingredients:

1	medium cabbage
3	medium carrots
2–3	garlic cloves, peeled
1	onion
1	thumb-sized piece of ginger, peeled
15 mL (1 tbsp)	unrefined sea salt
5 mL (1 tsp)	pepper (pre-ground or freshly crushed peppercorns)[1]

Equipment:

1	mixing container (e.g., large bowl or pot)
1	knife, hand grater, or electric food processor
2	1-litre (4-cup) wide-mouth mason jars
1	tight-fitting lid per jar

Remove the two outermost cabbage leaves and set aside (these will be used later). Shred the vegetables and put them into a large mixing bowl (I use my large soup pot). Add the sea salt. Add ground black pepper or crushed peppercorns, to taste. Mix this up. Allow the salted vegetable mixture to sit for 20–30 minutes to let some of the cabbage's juices draw out. Knead the mixture. Some people, especially those with strength issues, skip the kneading altogether by simply adding saltwater (5 mL or 1 teaspoon salt to 250 mL or 1 cup water) over the batch. You can get extra leverage by placing the mixing bowl on the floor and rocking your whole body over your hands. If very little juice is developing within a full minute of kneading, add another 7.5 mL (½ tablespoon) of salt and continue kneading. Continue kneading until firmly pressing your flat palms onto the batch draws juices over much of your hands. Pack the mixture into jar(s), leaving at least 5 cm (2 inches) of air space at the top. Press the veggie mixture down, to get most of the air pockets out. Juice will rise to the top. Press pieces of whole cabbage leaves on top, right to the edges of the jar (even going up the sides of the jar a bit) to "seal" in the top layer of shredded veggies. The juice will rise up over much of the leaves. Close the jar lid tightly.

Place the jar in an area away from direct sunlight that maintains a temperature of 18°C–24°C (64°F–75°F). If using an Excalibur® dehydrator, set the machine to its lowest temperature point (i.e., barely "on"). In mine, this brings the temperature to 20°C–21°C (68°F–70°F), which works perfectly. After four to seven days (four if the temperature is closer to 24°C or 75°F; seven if the

---

[1] Can add more to taste.

temperature is closer to 18°C–21°C or 68°F–70°F), move the unopened jar into the fridge.

When to open and eat it? For several years, people doing GAPS have followed instructions to use a batch after just four to seven days of countertop fermentation. Many of us have had great success with this. However, some people may do best with a longer fermentation (the batch will also get yummier as it ages either opened or unopened in the fridge). If you are concerned you may react to a younger ferment, do this: After the four to seven days of countertop fermentation, move the unopened jar to a cool place, such as your cellar or your fridge. Leave it there for four to nine weeks before using.

When you wish to start eating a batch, open the jar and remove (throw out) the top cabbage leaves. If there is fuzziness on top, this may be one of several things. A neutral coloured texture may simply be "bloom." Some people throw out this layer and eat the rest of the jar's contents. Personally, I mix mine in and eat the whole batch. Fuzziness with a distinct colour or any other concerning characteristic may be mould. In this case, the whole batch should be thrown out.

When you are ready, enjoy the contents. Keep the remainder of the batch in the closed jar in the fridge. The fermented vegetables can be eaten any time from this point forward, but will continue to deepen in flavour over subsequent weeks.

Yogurt

Many people will skip yogurt and move directly to kefir, which requires less fuss and equipment (but kefir's healing properties can overwhelm a body in the early stages of healing). Those who cannot yet tolerate the healing power of kefir, those who specifically enjoy the texture or flavour of yogurt, or those who want to gain from the benefits of sour cream, may use the following steps (any other yogurt recipe that incorporates GAPS' fermentation temperatures and durations is also acceptable).

- **Equipment:** Until you find a consistently effective method of maintaining your desired temperature, be sure to check the temperature of the yogurt itself (not just the surrounding air) throughout your chosen process. If underheated, the bacteria will not be able to activate and propagate. Overheated, the beneficial bacteria can be killed off, resulting in more lactose than a person's body can cope with. It is essential to maintain the recommended fermentation temperature for at least 24–29 hours (an even longer fermentation time of 36 hours is helpful for people especially sensitive to lactose). There are several ways to do this.

o The cheapest approach is to temporarily replace your oven light with a 60-watt bulb, then adjust the door gap regularly (it is critical to replace the bulb upon completion of the fermentation, otherwise when you next turn the oven on, the bulb could shatter!). I did try this initially with much frustration and poor success in terms of maintaining the temperature for longer than an hour at a time.

o Some have great success using a crockpot, a jar wrapped in towels and set inside an insulated container, or a jar wrapped in a heating pad. Those of us who maintain very cool homes have been delighted with the Excalibur® dehydrator, which allows sensitive temperature adjustments (you can also make jerky, crackers, and fruit leather in it). The Yogourmet Multi yogurt maker is also commonly used, but cannot maintain the temperature for the required number of hours. Some folks have remedied this by plugging the Yogourmet into a lamp cord dimmer (available at hardware and lighting stores) and adjusting the dimmer until the desired temperature is reached (mark that setting for next time).

- **Starter:** You can use a commercial (powder) starter, plain commercial yogurt, or your own yogurt (or yogurt whey) from a previous homemade batch. If your own yogurt or whey stops working at any point, start again with a portion of commercial yogurt or commercial powder.

- **Milk:** Non-pasteurized, non-homogenized, full-fat milk is ideal. More people tolerate goat's milk than cow's milk, but the reverse may be true for some individuals. Thus, raw, organic goat milk is a great place to start. In my experience, goat's milk results in a tarter product than cow's milk, but not necessarily a thinner one as is commonly claimed. If goat, raw, or organic milk is not available, any milk can be tested and will likely be as well tolerated as any other.

Directions:

Note: Raw milk can be used heated, as follows, or unheated (heating it will produce a more consistent texture).

Stirring occasionally, bring 1 litre (4 cups) of milk to 82°C (180°F) (i.e., just approaching a boil). Do not bring to a boil. Let cool to 20°C–25°C (68°F–77°F). Add starter. This may be commercial starter (add the amount directed by the manufacturer) or 80 mL (⅓ cup) of commercial yogurt or of a previously homemade batch of yogurt or whey. Stir to completely dissolve (a hand whisk works well). Pour into containers, such as canning jars, and cover with a lid or a towel secured by an elastic band. Set the containers in a place that will bring the liquid (not just the surrounding air) back up to 35°C–43°C (95°F–110°F) and then maintain this temperature for 24–36 hours (36 hours is helpful for those people especially sensitive to lactose). After this period, the yogurt can be eaten, but if you want a firmer, thicker product, follow these additional steps before disturbing (i.e., shaking, stirring, or eating from) the batch: Very gently, move the containers of undisturbed yogurt to the fridge. Leave the containers in the fridge for eight hours to set, then use freely.

The yogurt can be refrigerated and used for up to several months. After three weeks, its population of beneficial bacteria may begin to decrease slightly. Freezing the yogurt may kill much of the bacteria, so this is not recommended. However, yogurt that has been frozen would remain a lactose-free dairy and would be acceptable as a non-probiotic dairy for GAPS.

Sour Cream (Crème Fraîche)

Follow the directions for *Yogurt*, but use cream instead of milk and stir the thicker product more frequently during the heating process. For sour cream, raw cream will provide a consistent texture even without being heated first, so heating is optional.

Kefir

Dairy kefir is a thick drink rich in friendly bacteria and yeasts (these yeasts are suitable for an anti-*Candida* diet). Its consistency may vary from almost as thin as milk to nearly as thick as yogurt (this will vary throughout the year). I use goat's milk for mine, and it results in a product very similar in taste and texture to commercial buttermilk.

Hydrated kefir "grains" (not grains at all) are blobs that often look like tiny cauliflower florets and feel a bit like gummy bears. The kefir grains are used as a starter to ferment dairy. When people say they are drinking kefir, they are referring to the liquid created. However, it is fine and very health-giving to also eat the grains themselves.

Because it is such a powerfully healing food, be sure to start with just 5 mL (1 teaspoon) or less on the first day and work up slowly, perhaps increasing by just another 5 mL (1 teaspoon) once a week initially. Taking too much too soon can cause intense detox or die-off symptoms.

Following are two methods for making kefir. Any other kefir recipe that incorporates GAPS' fermentation temperatures and durations is also acceptable.

Kefir, Dairy (Simple Version)

When I first started making kefir, I wanted a lot of information plus detailed instructions, which I offer subsequently. Through experimentation and eventual familiarity with kefir, I learned that some steps (e.g., stirring or shaking every eight hours) were not necessary. My process became much simpler and is now as follows:

To 1 litre (4 cups) of milk, add 15 mL (1 tablespoon) of dairy kefir grains. Cover the container with a paper towel or cloth towel. Set anywhere in the house away from direct sunlight and let the kefir sit. In temperatures warmer than 21°C (70°F), eight hours may be enough to achieve kefir, but for GAPS purposes, we ferment it for at least 24 hours. In temperatures cooler than 19°C (66°F), leave it for 36 hours (longer is fine. Only because I don't get around to the final step, I often leave mine out for one to three weeks!).

Stir the kefir and then pour it into a plastic colander with a container placed below it. Allow the kefir to drain. The grains will remain behind in the colander. Keep 15 mL (1 tablespoon) of the grains for a subsequent batch (a new batch can be started immediately, or the grains can be saved in a bit of milk or kefir, either covered or uncovered, in the fridge or freezer). Grains not needed for subsequent batches can be eaten (dosed the same as the kefir itself) or offered to others who need them. The kefir can be enjoyed immediately or refrigerated indefinitely.

Kefir, Dairy (Detailed Instructions)

Developed in partnership with Patty Donovan

Materials Required

- Glass jar(s)
- Paper or cloth towel and elastic band
- Strainer
- Dairy kefir grains
- Milk from any animal

FERMENTATION TEMPERATURE

The ideal temperature for kefir fermentation is 20°C–25°C (68°F–77°F). This will create a successful ferment within 24–36 hours. Cooler is fine, but the cooler it is, the longer the ferment will take. In warmer temperatures, kefir will culture very rapidly. In an environment warmer than 25°C (77°F), you may want to culture it for 12 hours on the counter and then 12 hours in the fridge. According to a wintertime experiment in my cool house, an Excalibur dehydrator set to its lowest possible spot on the temperature dial will generally run 20°C–23°C (68°F–73°F).

Cover: The paper or cloth towel held by an elastic band will provide a cover for your jar that allows air through while keeping dust, etc., out.

Strainer and other tools: Some say kefir should never come in contact with any metal. Dominic Anfiteatro ("Dom"), a kefir guru, feels it is fine to use non-reactive materials (e.g., stainless steel) for tools the kefir is in brief contact with, such as the strainer, spoons, and so on (glass is preferable for the fermentation and storage). However, many people choose to use plastic or silicone tools.

Milk: Raw milk is preferable, but not everyone has access to this or can afford it. Organic is also preferable, but pasteurized (preferably non-homogenized) milk will work well, too. If at all possible, avoid ultra-pasteurized: it will still make a great kefir, but the effects of ultra-pasteurization may result in a kefir less easy for the body to process. In my experience, goat's milk results in a tarter product than cow's milk, but not necessarily a thinner one as is commonly claimed.

All materials must be truly clean of substances other than the ingredients used. However, it is fine to reuse the fermentation jar for several batches in a row without washing it between uses—this will support the growth and maintenance of the grains and kefiran (a soft, jelly-like goop that eventually develops around the grains and which is extremely health-giving).

Steps
1. **Obtaining Grains**. Freeze-dried kefir starter can be purchased in health food stores and online. This starter will not reproduce so you will continually have to rebuy it. Freeze-dried starter is less effective than whole kefir grains because it has only about ten strains of bacteria and yeast to the live grains' 35 strains. To obtain whole dairy kefir grains, post a request to your online GAPS support list or look online for someone offering them. Dom, the kefir guru mentioned earlier, hosts a Yahoo Group (http://groups.yahoo.com/group/Kefir_making/) through which he can provide grains. Have your supplies ready for when your grains arrive. Be prepared to purchase some milk upon their arrival.
2. **Upon Receiving Your Grains (Dehydrated or Fresh)**.
    a) Dehydrated Grains (hard and yellow): Dehydrated grains will need to be run through several batches to be revived, possibly over two or three weeks.
        i.   Rinse the kefir grains with fresh milk (not water).
        ii.   Put the grains into a jar.
        iii.   Pour just enough fresh milk to cover the grains.
        iv.   Cover the jar with a towel secured by an elastic band.

      v.   Set the jar in an environment of 20°C–25°C (68°F–77°F).

      vi.   Every one to two days, dispose of the milk (but not the grains) and add a fresh supply of milk.

      vii. Repeat this process until the grains are fluffy, white, and soft. At that point, rinse them once more with fresh milk and then proceed to the instructions under "Fresh Grains," following.

  b) Fresh Grains (soft, white blobs)

      i.   Into a quart (1-litre) jar, place approximately 15 mL (1 tablespoon) of grains.

      ii.   Over the grains, pour approximately 1 litre (4 cups) of milk (with time and experimentation, you may find that your grains desire a different ratio and that's fine).

      iii. Cover the jar with a towel secured by an elastic band.

      iv. Set the jar in an environment of 20°C–25°C (68°F–77°F).

      v.   After approximately eight hours, remove the towel and gently stir the contents. This will help the milk to stay mixed with the grains. Replace the towel.

      vi.   After 24 hours or so (12 hours in warm weather), look at the sides of the jar. Are there tiny rivulets snaking down the sides? These indicate the beginning of whey separation and are one indication of readiness. Do you see a slight separation of curds and whey? This is another sign of readiness. Does the product smell yeasty (like pizza dough) and sour (like yogurt)? These are also signs of readiness. Occasionally, a first batch will have an "off" odour. Although probably safe, you may want to discard this batch, keeping only the grains. It may take several batches for the grains to acclimatize to your house and milk source. At the signs of readiness, set a toothpick vertically into the kefir. If the kefir holds the toothpick up, it's ready. Depending on the ambient temperature, your first few batches may require longer than 24 hours, and even up to 36 hours. If a batch appears ready after just 8–12 hours, feel free to move it into the fridge for the remainder of its fermentation time.

3. **Separating the kefir from the kefir grains**. When the kefir is ready, you need to separate the kefir from the kefir grains.

  a) Strainer Method: Set a strainer over a jar or bowl. Into the strainer, pour the entire contents of the jar. You might need to let the kefir drip out over several minutes, or stir the strainer's contents to help the liquid move through.

b) Hand Method: If your kefir is too thick for a strainer, wash your hands well then pull the grains out (the grains will feel firm and not fall apart; the curds, on the other hand, will fall apart).

Except as noted, never rinse the grains. Simply begin the whole cycle again, starting at Step 2(b) where 1 litre (4 cups) of milk is poured over 15 mL (1 tablespoon) of grains in a quart jar.

4. **Preserve a Back-up Batch**. Sometimes, bad things happen to good grains. For those times, it is helpful to have a back-up batch of grains. Once your grains start increasing in size or number, freeze or dehydrate some.

a) To Freeze: Put the grains in ice cube trays or in small jars, barely covered with milk. Dom recommends that grains spend no longer than six months in the freezer. However, some have reported success reconstituting frozen grains after more than two years.

b) To Dehydrate: Dehydrated grains can successfully be reconstituted after a year or more.

    i. Rinse grains in chlorine-free water.

    ii. Pat dry.

    iii. Lay grains out on linen or paper towels.

    iv. Cover grains with another towel.

    v. Every day, agitate them (i.e., move them around a bit).

    vi. Depending on room temperature and humidity, drying usually takes three to five days. When the grains are completely dry (i.e., hard, small, and yellowish), put them into a baggie and store in the refrigerator.

Secondary Ferment

Kefir uses up most of milk's lactose. However, if you are concerned about any remaining sugar content, you can do a secondary ferment. After straining the grains out of a batch that has fermented for 24–36 hours, set the kefir out at the usual fermentation temperatures for one more day or in the fridge for five to six days. The resulting kefir will be very tart. People put off by tartness might use it in a smoothie with fruits, for example.

Kefir Issues

1. **Grains not Growing**

a) Use milk from antibiotic-free animals.

b) Make sure your tools are dry and free of any chlorine from tap water.

c) Rinse the grains in chlorine-free filtered water and then rest them in plain organic yogurt for 24 hours before using the grains again.

2. **Kefir Smells "Strange"**

a) Kefir's characteristic scent is "yeasty" (similar to pizza dough). This is normal and usually not a problem. However, a very strong yeasty scent can be balanced via a yogurt rest: Rinse the grains in chlorine-free filtered water and then rest them in plain organic yogurt for 24 hours. This "yogurt rest" will restore the balance between the bacteria and yeast.

b) Sometimes kefir will have a strong chemical smell (such as that used in varnish, etc). Kefir produces multiple aromatic compounds as it ferments. Long ferments are more likely to produce these at a noticeable level. The kefir is still safe to drink.

c) If the kefir smells disgusting, there is a possibility that it is contaminated. Try the yogurt rest mentioned above. If the nasty smell persists in a subsequent batch, throw out the kefir and the grains and start with new grains (this is where your back-up batch comes in!).

d) If mould (green, grey, fuzzy) ever forms, throw your kefir and grains away. Again, this is where your back-up batch can come in.

3. **Grains Get Large and Flat**

This is normal. It occurs occasionally and is nothing to worry about. It usually means you have too many grains for the quantity of milk you are using. Break the grains up and increase the milk-to-grain ratio (i.e., more milk or fewer grains).

4. **Grains Very Large and/or Slow Growing**

Break the grains into smaller pieces. This will rapidly increase their growth rate.

5. **Storing Grains**

You will be building your dose of kefir very slowly at the start. Thus, a small amount of kefir will go a long way, and you will not need large batches. You may also need to back off on kefir production from time to time. At these points, the method for storing kefir grains is very helpful (repeat for as many weeks as you wish):

a) Without rinsing them first, put the grains into a jar.

b) Pour over the grains just enough fresh milk to cover.

c) Once a week, dispose of this milk (but not the grains) and add fresh milk.

6. **Too Many Grains**

When you have more grains than you need for regular ferments and a back-up supply, you can eat the grains or offer them out to folks in need of some.

Kefir, Dairy-Free

For GAPS, it is fine to make kefir from any liquid, including non-dairy ones such as coconut water or sweetened water. Dairy grains can be used to make non-dairy kefir, but dairy grains should be rinsed thoroughly before use in a non-dairy liquid, as well as rested in milk after use. If you will be regularly making non-dairy kefir, invest in grains suited for non-dairy kefir (i.e., "water grains") by requesting these from someone on one of the e-mail support lists or elsewhere.

Before making non-dairy kefir, review the instructions for *Dairy Kefir* as this will give you a sense of the overall process and considerations. For non-dairy kefir, follow these directions: Into a glass jar, put 60 mL (¼ cup) of water kefir grains and 1 litre (4 cups) of sweetened liquid, such as coconut water. Cover the opening of the jar with paper towel or a cloth and secure it with an elastic band. Let it sit in a warm area for 36–48 hours. Strain out the grains. Refrigerate. Enjoy any time. Again, any type of kefir will be very powerful. Start with a teaspoon or less and work up slowly.

Fermented Whey and Cream Cheese

To obtain fermented whey, do the following: Pour homemade yogurt or homemade kefir into a nut milk bag (available at most health food stores), a large piece of cheesecloth, or similar material. With a container underneath it, hang the bag from a cupboard doorknob. Alternatively, line a colander with cheesecloth and set the colander over a bowl, or drape a nut milk bag or cloth over a container, with room below the bag for dripping, and secure it with an elastic band. Allow several hours for dripping. The relatively clear liquid that drips out is fermented whey. Stored in a clean jar in the fridge, the whey can be used as is, as a probiotic source or starter, or diluted with water or juice as a probiotic drink. If making whey to use as a starter (e.g., for the *Fermented Fish* recipe) long before yogurt is introduced into your diet, you can refrigerate the yogurt for several weeks.

Left until all the whey is dripped or squeezed out, the yogurt or kefir remaining in the bag can be used as a soft cottage cheese, a thicker yogurt, or a spreadable cream cheese.

Fermented Fish

By the time a person reaches the point in Intro in which fermented fish is introduced, they are usually a good two weeks or so into Intro. Thus, for most people this is a suitable time to test this lower-allergen dairy (and it is usually well tolerated). The following instructions are adapted from recipes provided by Dr. Campbell-McBride.

Ingredients:

4	sardines, herring, or mackerel
125 mL (½ cup)	whey from yogurt or kefir
7.5 mL (½ tbsp)	salt (per 500 mL water)
15 mL (1 tbsp)	black peppercorns, freshly crushed
5	bay leaves
5 mL (1 tsp)	coriander seeds, freshly crushed

To prevent the ingestion of parasites, you can use fish that has been commercially frozen for at least two weeks (home freezers do not typically sustain temperatures cold enough to kill parasites). Your fishmonger can tell you which fish options are suitable for using in a raw fish dish. Descale and debone each fish. Cut the head off and clean the belly out. Cut into bite-size pieces. Put the fish pieces into a glass jar. Add black peppercorns, bay leaves, and coriander seeds. Separately, dissolve 7.5 mL (½ tablespoon) salt into 500 mL (2 cups) water. To the salt water, add the whey. Pour the liquid over the fish. If the fish is not quite covered, add more of the solution or plain, non-chlorinated water. Close the jar lid tightly. Let it ferment for three to five days at room temperature, then refrigerate. Serve within three weeks, with fresh dill and some chopped red onion.

Beans, Proper Preparation

The following applies to dried beans (white navy, haricot, and lima), lentils, and split peas. Soak the dried beans, lentils, or split peas in water (with no additives) for 12–24 hours. Drain. Rinse well under running water. Cover with a new batch of water. Add 125 mL (½ cup) of whey per 1 litre (4 cups) of water. Set out at room temperature (20°C–25°C or 68°F–77°F). Leave to ferment. In an environment warmer than "room temperature," soak for just two days; in a cooler environment, soak three to five days. Rinse well. Proceed with cooking. After sufficient healing, you may be able to skip the fermentation (i.e., whey-inclusive) step and use the beans, etc., after just the initial 12–24 hour soak.

CHAPTER 16

RECIPES: MORE ESSENTIALS

Replenishing Drinks

A replenishing drink that offers fluid as well as minerals and/or carbohydrates has many purposes. Depending on the drink's ingredients, it can rehydrate a person who has had diarrhea or vomiting, flush out toxins without depleting the body of key minerals, add carbohydrates to reduce the degree and effects of ketosis, trigger appetite in a person who temporarily has none, or entice a child to drink when they will not otherwise do so.

A replenishing drink can be natural, homemade, or commercially produced. It may be as simple as 15 mL (1 tablespoon) of apple cider vinegar added to 250 mL (1 cup) of water. This can help a person to feel balanced, invigorated, and well. Other excellent sources of balancing minerals include meat broth with salt added, bananas, breast milk, kefir, citrus fruits, and so on. However, in early Intro, we generally avoid fruits and even excellent dairy, such as kefir.

Meat broth with sea salt added is an excellent base for one's early program, but when additional support is needed, an additional replenishing drink may prove very helpful in cases of nausea, lethargy, loss of appetite, or a general feeling of unwellness. A cupful can help put one back on track and reinstate an appetite for broth, meat, fats, and/or vegetables. In addition, some people see better overall health when they incorporate an electrolyte drink every day. You can search online for a homemade electrolyte drink recipe or oral rehydration solution. Most of these involve very specific ratios of pure water, baking soda, sea salt, honey, and lemon juice (or another source of potassium). Coconut water (not coconut milk) is a natural source of electrolytes and is also GAPS-friendly. However, coconut water can trigger diarrhea in some people. If this is true for you, discontinue its use. Health food stores sell powdered mixes, using ingredients of varying qualities. These may be suitable in a rehydration emergency; otherwise, try to use options which include only GAPS-friendly ingredients. On the *Support for You* page at GAPSguide.com, there is a link to several online recipes for electrolyte drinks and oral rehydration solutions.

It is quite common for children to refuse food for three to five days in early Intro, and a replenishing drink during that period can help prevent major problems, such as dehydration. Some sources express a need for due caution when it comes to preparing and providing homemade electrolyte drinks to children under the age of 12 years, so look for one that is appropriate to your child's age. A baby or child with access to breast milk can be well-served throughout a period of discomfort or imbalance by nursing more frequently. When a child is very lethargic or nauseated, a small amount of fruit juice heavily diluted with water, or 80 mL (⅓ cup) of frozen banana chunks, or a cup of purified water with 5 mL (1 teaspoon) of honey, a pinch of salt, and a squeeze of fresh orange or lemon can help. Whether the age-appropriate replenishing drink is a GAPS broth or ferment, based on a recipe sourced from the Internet, or purchased from the health food store, it must not become one's primary "food" or a food replacement. That is, to prevent or resolve dehydration, the drink should be approached as the medically necessary medicine that it is, but when dehydration is not a concern, the replenishing drink can be used in a quantity just sufficient to stimulate appetite, relieve some of the sensation of die-off, or quickly infuse the body with enough carbohydrates to reduce the discomfort of ketosis. In these cases, the replenishing drink should be used in moderation and kept secondary to "real" food—a child's initial period of food refusal notwithstanding.

Homemade Fat (Lard or Tallow)

This makes up to 2.5 litres (10 cups).

This method is just one of many approaches available to you. You might start with these fats and this approach, and shortly move on to any other, such as using a crockpot, different fats, or the wet-rendering method. There are many tutorials available on the Internet, many with excellent photographs depicting the process.

When fat is initially drawn from an animal, it is attached to other elements (e.g., meat and connective tissue) which can cause the fat to go rancid. In rendering fat, we withdraw everything but the pure fat itself, which allows it to become stable for storage and for high-temperature cooking.

From your butcher or farmer, request approximately 2.3 kilograms (5 pounds) of lard (pig) or suet (cow or sheep). Alternatively, take the raw, firm, solid fat from any animal you are processing yourself, remove any remaining non-fat, and freeze it until you have collected about 2.3 kilograms (5 pounds).

Set aside time for the remaining steps. Especially the first few times, the trimming can take a good while, while the melting will always take a good hour or two.

Whatever the source, ensure all meat and bloody connective tissue—everything but the fat—is trimmed off. Blood and meat will ruin the rendering process.

Cut the fat into cubes. If you want the process to go faster, or you want to potentially gain more product, freeze these cubes of fat for approximately one to two hours—long enough for them to firm up but not long enough to fully freeze—then run them through your food processor on "shred."

Place the pieces in a roasting pan (for the oven) or in a heavy-bottomed pot (for the stovetop). Set your oven to 120°C (250°F) or set your stove to medium-low. It is critical to use a low temperature over a longer period of time. You want to gently melt the fat—not boil or even simmer. Monitor the process, stirring occasionally to unstick any pieces from the cookware. Inside the pot, cracklings (pieces of fried skin) may develop. When all the fat has melted, remove the pan or pot from the heat. Allow everything to cool and remove the cracklings with a slotted spoon.

> ## IMPORTANT
> Do not pour hot fat into glass jars. They may break, putting you at risk of injury! Allow the contents to cool for a few minutes, but proceed with the next step before the fat cools enough to solidify.

Drape a sieve or cheesecloth into the mouth of a jar (or use a funnel if the jar mouth is small), anchoring the cloth with an elastic band. Pour the warm (not hot) fat through the sieve or cheesecloth into the jar. Close the jar with a tight-fitting lid while the fat is still warm.

While liquid, the fat will be a light amber or golden colour. As it cools, the fat will become solid and white.

Because different fats have different uses, label the jar by the type of fat. The rendered fat will keep in the fridge for months and in the freezer indefinitely. Keep what you need for the week in your fridge or on your counter. Use the fat to cook or bake with, add it to completed soups, or use it as a spread in place of butter.

Broth

Broth is a staple in GAPS. Ideally, we will have several cups of it per day during Intro, whether on its own or in soups or sauces, and at least 250 mL (1 cup) per day after that for health maintenance. Broth is chock-full of minerals and super healing for the gut. Chicken broth is especially soothing for gut inflammation. As it is so nourishing, broth tends to eliminate cravings, and it also makes an excellent restorative drink.

With sea salt added, mineral-rich broth can be sipped (hot or cold) from a mug, or used as a soup base (with or without additional water, depending on how hearty it is). It can be reduced (i.e., simmered until the excess water evaporates) into a sauce. The sauce can then be cooked with, poured or drizzled over a dish, used as a dip, and so on.

Broth can be made from any animal. Animals, like humans, contain that which they eat, drink, and are exposed to environmentally; therefore, eating from various animals ensures you get the widest range of nutrients as determined by each animal's environment and diet. Meat, bones, and joints from wild or pastured, grass-fed, free-range, chemical-free animals are preferable.

With experimentation, you may find you are sensitive to one type of broth, but do well with another. As with all GAPS foods, experimentation may be the only way to find out which broths you might be reactive to. Test each type (e.g., sheep versus bison) separately. If you find you are reactive to one or two, continue to use as wide a variety as possible of any you tolerate. Experiment with meat and bones from sheep, salmon, chicken, cow, buffalo, turkey, and so on. If a number of broths seem problematic, try wild options, such as pheasant, deer, or quail—the more uncommon the better. Fish from fresh water (e.g., clean lakes and rivers) is good. Fish from the deep sea is better than that from coastal areas. Although tuna is mentioned in the list of permitted foods, Dr. Campbell-McBride recommends that we generally avoid large carnivorous fish such as tuna and shark. Vary all sources of meat and fish as much and as often as possible.

To make a broth, you can cook a whole chicken or whole fish, animal parts such as chicken backs or turkey legs, or meaty bones and joints requested from your local butcher or the grocery store meat counter. Many health food stores can special order meaty bones or joints from grass-fed, free-range, chemical-free animals. It is the bones, joints, and soft tissues that are critical; the meat is secondary.

Fill the pot so the meaty bones or joints will still be immersed after some evaporation occurs. The more water you use in relation to bone mass, the less concentrated the broth will be; the less water you use, the more concentrated it will be. For a lighter broth, more water can also be added after the simmer; for a more concentrated liquid, broth can be "reduced" (see the recipe for *Sauce/Dip*). Concentrated broth can be reconstituted by adding water at any point during or after preparation.

Meat Broth vs. Bone Broth

In GAPS we refer to "meat broth" and "bone broth." What is the difference between the two? Meat broth uses meat-on-bone and/or meat-on-joints and is simmered for a relatively short period of time (one to three hours), just long enough to make the meat safe for eating and the marrow accessible. Meat broth is highly nourishing and triggers reactions in relatively few people, so I recommend you start your program with this.

Bone broth, on the other hand, does not have to include meat, and the bones are simmered for a much longer period (up to 48 hours). Bone broth is even more nourishing than meat broth, but it can trigger reactions in some people, especially children and sensitive adults who are in the early stages of healing. Although it can be included right from the start of your program if tolerated, I recommend that you test the long-simmered bone broth any time after completing Intro.

Eating Broth

Broth can be taken on its own, as part of a soup, as a sauce, etc. For children or adults not keen on plain broth, here are some ideas:

1. Serve the broth as part of a soup or thick stew, rather than having it on its own (blending a soup or stew also makes these dishes more acceptable to many children).
2. Simmer the broth until much of its water content evaporates, leaving behind a thicker substance (a "reduction sauce"). The longer you let it simmer, the thicker it gets. I like to drizzle this reduction sauce over this Guide's *Shepherd's Pie* recipe, for example.
3. Cook vegetables in broth. One option: Add sliced vegetables to the broth and let them simmer uncovered in the broth until much of the water content evaporates and your veggies are resting in a warm, thick coating of flavour (this dish's flavour is akin to a stir-fry).
4. Pour broth into or onto any other savoury dish, like mashed cauliflower, lentil-mushroom pizzas, etc. (for these dishes, I especially like the broth with ghee, salt, and pepper added).
5. Several children on our support lists will take warm (not hot) broth happily if presented with a straw.
6. A chef and GAPS veteran, Justine, suggests setting things in the cooked down broth. She gives headcheese and souse as examples, but notes that one can just as well chop up cooked meat and veggies and set these in any gelatin-rich broth that is cooked down enough. Her family eats slices of this by hand.
7. One little girl only likes her broth when it is mixed with cod liver oil, so her mom adds the daily dose to 80 mL (⅓ cup) of broth.

8. Another mom, whose child would not take the broth in any form, explained to her daughter that her tummy was sick and that broth was her medicine. The mom filled a syringe-type medicine dropper and squirted the broth into her daughter's mouth, teaspoon by teaspoon. Over time, the little girl worked progressively up to cup-size servings.

9. At least one mom has had success by adding a small amount of fresh carrot and apple juice to her child's cup of broth.

10. Offer a reward (e.g., a star on a chart or a preferred GAPS food) for every sip of broth or bite of broth-drenched vegetables or meat.

If you love to drink broth by the mugful, that's wonderful! However, if you cannot stand it that way, whatever way you do get it in is just fine. Many children and adults have healed fantastically without a large daily dose, so don't stress too much about this!

Finally, various sources on the Internet offer wonderful information about broth. One of my favourite articles on broth is "Traditional Bone Broth in Modern Health and Disease" by Dr. Allison Siebecker for the *Townsend Letter for Doctors & Patients* (http://www.townsendletter.com/FebMarch2005/broth0205.htm).

Meat Broth

Use a whole fish, a whole chicken, or meaty bones and joints from any animal. When requesting bones, ask your butcher to cut the bones horizontally or into small chunks to expose the marrow. Put the raw, meaty bones and joints into a pot large enough to contain them. Fill the pot with water. Add some freshly crushed black peppercorns to infuse the broth with more digestive aid. Put the lid on. Bring to barely a boil. Skim the foam from the top. Put the lid back on and reduce to barely a simmer. Simmer the contents for one to three hours. Turn off the heat and add sea salt to taste. Broth should smell meaty, but mild. With sea salt added, the broth should have a light, delicious flavour. If it smells or tastes "off" (some people have reported this issue to me, but I don't know why it happens), throw it out. While the broth is still warm and fluid, remove and set aside the bones, joints, and meat. Use a sieve to ensure all small bones are withdrawn. The meat, and everything soft within or surrounding the bones and joints, can be eaten or saved (see the *Pâté* recipe). The bones can be frozen for bone broth later in your program or discarded.

Enjoy as much of the broth as you wish right away—as a drink from a mug or as a base for your next soup or sauce. The rest can be refrigerated for up to 1 week, or frozen for 2-3 months. Tip: Freeze in portions sufficient for one soup or 1 week so that you can easily thaw just what you need rather than having to attack a large block with a sledgehammer!

Upon cooling, the broth may or may not have a thin or thick layer of fat on top and/or gelatin throughout. This is fine. Various factors, including the type and cut of meat and bone, etc., will determine what the end product looks like. All batches will offer strong healing qualities. If you cannot yet tolerate fat, let the broth cool, remove the fat from the top, freeze it, and enjoy the mineral-rich broth itself. Over time, include more and more of the fat in your meals.

Bone Broth

When meat broth is well tolerated, you can test bone broth. For bone broth, you can use bones and joints that were previously cooked, such as with a chicken soup or roast, or bones and joints that have not been previously cooked. The bones and joints can have meat on them or not. I usually wait until I have about 1 kg (2.2 pounds) of bones. Initially I kept a container in the freezer, throwing in fish tails, chicken bones, etc., until I had about a kilogram of bones, tails, and other pieces. Recently I have been purchasing bones, with or without meat on them, from butchers.

If purchasing bones from a butcher, ask her to smash or cut the bones to expose the marrow. Put the bones and joints into a pot. If tolerated, add approximately 15 mL (1 tablespoon) of apple cider vinegar to the pot; this will help draw minerals from the soup bones. Fill the pot with water. Simmer 12–36 hours. If you plan to simmer for over 12 hours, expect 2.5–5 cm or 1–2 inches of water to evaporate. Bones simmered for a very long time may fall apart. It is normal for small bones to become so brittle that they disintegrate in one's hand. A sieve will allow you to remove even the smallest pieces of bone (very soft bones can be eaten and provide much nutrition). Add salt. Enjoy as you would meat broth.

Pâté

From a pot of broth, remove the meat, bones, and joints (use a strainer for very small bones) and set them on a clean surface. From the meat, bones, and joints—inside, outside, all around—remove any of the soft stuff (e.g., tissue, marrow, fat, skin, and so on). You can eat any of this if you are ready to do so. Otherwise, put the soft stuff into a container, add some meat, salt, and any spices you like, blend it, and label it "pâté." You can enjoy it immediately as a spread or dip, or you can refrigerate or freeze it.

Sauce/Dip

Into a pot put any broth. With no lid on it, allow it to simmer. Over the minutes or hours, more and more of the broth's water content will evaporate, turning the broth thicker and thicker. (From the appropriate points in Intro, any herbs and spices can also be added to a sauce or dip.) When the desired thickness is achieved, use this "reduction" as a sauce or dip for meat strips, vegetables, etc. Note: Using the same approach, tomatoes can be cooked, blended, and then reduced to create a tomato sauce or dip or, with additional ingredients, ketchup.

Ginger Tea

Take a piece of whole, raw ginger about the size of your thumb. Slice it very thinly. Add it to a pot of water. Simmer for 20 minutes. Taste. If it is too strong, simply add more water. In early Intro, it is fine (but not necessary) to add 5 mL (1 teaspoon) or less of honey to each cup.

Nuts and Seeds

Nuts and seeds are something to watch carefully on GAPS. Many people love the flavours, textures, and versatility they bring to the program. Nuts and seeds are indeed tasty, are available almost everywhere, and are very portable. Most exciting of all for GAPSters is that they make wonderful flours, allowing for the reintroduction of a more typical muffin, bread, or cookie. When preparing to introduce nuts and seeds, it is important to pay attention to proportions. Nuts and seeds are a nutritional powerhouse, but in GAPS they should remain a dietary enhancement, not a foundation. Most of our meals and snacks should still be made of marrow, gelatin, fats, eggs, meats, ferments, and vegetables.

Many people (my son and me included) struggle with nuts and seeds for some time. These foods have enzyme inhibitors inherent to them that can challenge digestion in their as is state. Early on, commercial almond flour felt like a rock sitting at the bottom of my stomach. In my son, the same product triggered mushy stools. After various experiments (e.g., commercially prepared nut butters, unsoaked nuts, and commercial nut flours), I found that early in GAPS, preparing nuts and seeds by soaking was critically important. Even after several months, my son and I were still not able to digest very well the amounts of commercial almond or coconut flours we were tempted to use, so we continued to rely on soaking away the enzyme inhibitors. After about nine months on GAPS, we were each able to have approximately 125 mL (½ cup) of commercial (i.e., unsoaked) almond flour once a week, without problem. Eventually, we experienced no noticeable issues with any nut or seed flour. (Soaking is still good practice; besides making the food more digestible in general, it also enhances the value of the food by making its nutrients more bioavailable.) Our approach to these foods was as follows:

Purchase and Basic Preparation

Labelling of nuts and seeds varies from country to country. Thus, it is difficult to determine which are actually organic and/or raw—simply select the best option you can manage. Try to purchase ones that are either refrigerated or in a high turnover location, so that they are as fresh as possible (even a small amount of mould is an issue for some GAPS bodies). Store them in your fridge or freezer.

When you are ready to prepare them, put 1 litre (4 cups) of nuts or seeds into a bowl, sprinkle 30 mL (2 tablespoons) of sea salt over them (to keep unwanted bacteria at bay and to activate the enzymes), add 2 L (8 cups) of water, cover the bowl with a towel (to keep dust and bugs out), and leave the bowl on a counter for 4–24 hours. Personally, I soak any nut or seed for variable amounts of time within this time frame, depending on my personal schedule. Dr. Campbell-McBride suggests 12 hours for any seed and 24 hours for any nut, if an intolerance indicates need. Other sources specify a different soaking time for each type of nut or seed. If you want to test whether varying soaking times helps you achieve better digestion, you can do an Internet search for a "seed soaking chart." Sunflower and sesame seeds will double their size, so they need lots of water (add more as needed throughout their soaking time). Nuts and seeds can also be fermented for further digestibility: To 1 litre (4 cups) of nuts, add 2 L (8 cups) of water and 125 mL (½ cup) of whey. Soak for 24 hours at room temperature (20°C–25°C or 68°F–77°F). Drain and rinse very well.

Eating, Mashing, and Dehydrating

- **Eating as is:** Soaked nuts and seeds are plump and still slightly chewy or crunchy. They are a nice treat and a fantastic source of nutrition. Store soaked-and-rinsed nuts in the fridge and eat them within one to three days. Alternatively, spread the soaked-and-rinsed nuts on a cookie sheet, freeze them, then bag them. Over time you can scoop out and thaw just the amount you need, eating them as is, or mashing or dehydrating them.

- **Mashing:** If you want to mash the nuts or seeds—whether smoothly into a "butter" or coarsely for use in pizza crust, burger patties, or nut bars—you can run them through a heavy-duty food processor (or the homogenizing function on a higher-end juicer) within three days of soaking (and refrigerating). The soaked nuts/seeds have a high moisture content and will often come out somewhere between a nut butter and a nut flour. Slowly drizzling in oil while churning will result in a creamier mixture. Refrigerate and eat, or freeze, the product within three days of the initial soaking.

- **Dehydrating or Making Flour:** If you want crunchy nuts or a nut flour, place the nuts into a dehydrator after soaking and rinsing, following its instructions. Alternatively, arrange the nuts in one layer on a cookie sheet and set it into an oven on its lowest possible temperature, turning the nuts regularly until they are dry throughout. For a nut flour, run very dry nuts through a food processor after dehydrating, pulsing attentively to avoid churning the nuts into a butter.

Nut Butter Pancakes/Crepes

Instructions based on a recipe by Dr. Campbell-McBride.

Ingredients:

500 mL (2 cups)	butternut squash, peeled, de-seeded, and cooked
2	eggs
30 mL (2 tbsp)	any animal fat
250 mL (1 cup)	nut[1] butter (preferably pre-soaked and rinsed)

Blend the butternut squash, eggs, nut butter, and 15 mL (1 tablespoon) of the fat together. If needed, add more squash or eggs as required to make a thin, porridge-like consistency. Heat a pan to medium and add the other 15 mL (1 tablespoon) of tolerated fat to the pan. For easier flipping, make smaller pancakes (at least three should fit in a pan). Fry the pancakes on one side and then the other, moving quickly so as not to burn them.

Basic Bread/Cake/Muffin

Adapted from *Gut and Psychology Syndrome* (9th edition).

Ingredients:

625 mL (2½ cups)	nut or seed flour (ground nuts or seeds)
60 mL (¼ cup)	softened fat (e.g., butter, coconut oil, goose fat, duck fat) or homemade yogurt/sour cream
3	eggs

Mix ingredients well. Adjust the proportions of each ingredient, as needed, to achieve a porridge-like consistency. Grease a baking pan and pour the mixture in. Bake at 150°C (300°F) for approximately one hour (for a bread loaf). The bread is ready when an inserted knife comes out clean. As you progress on the diet, variations (e.g., savoury spices or raisins) can be incorporated.

---

[1] Alternatively, you can use sunflower seeds that have been soaked for three days then mashed.

Early Intro Casserole with Meat Pieces

Feel free to use any GAPS-friendly meat/veggie casserole recipe from any source—there are lots online. Following is a very simple approach that is rich in liquid, thus especially suitable for early Intro. When this is tolerated, feel free to progress toward casserole recipes less rich in liquid and more toward the solid end of the casserole spectrum, such as the *Shepherd's Pie* recipe in this Guide.

Select any animal pieces with meat on bones (e.g., turkey legs or *osso bucco* steaks). If bones are cut, preferably lengthwise, more nutrients will be added to the resulting dish. Place meat pieces into a baking dish. Fill the baking pan with enough water to cover the meat as much as possible. Brush fat (e.g., duck fat) onto any parts of the meat that are not covered with water. Into the water, stir freshly crushed peppercorns, salt, and any fresh (not dried) herbs. (In later stages, dried herbs may also be used.) Set onto the middle shelf of the oven set at 150°C–160°C (300°F–320°F). After 1½ hours, add chopped garlic, onions, and mushrooms (or any other vegetables) to the surrounding water. After another 40 minutes, check for doneness and a safe meat temperature. If marrow has floated out of the bones (it will appear and taste similar to softened white butter), gently stir the marrow into the surrounding sauce. Remove the meat and veggies for eating immediately, and reserve any of the leftover liquid (broth) for use as a drink or soup base.

Shepherd's Pie

This recipe uses the Stage 4 stew as a base, so introduce it in Stage 4 or later. Make the *Beef Stew* recipe presented in this Guide. Separately, coarsely chop two medium-size heads of cauliflower, steam until soft, then blend with fat (e.g., ghee or duck fat) or broth, plus salt and pepper. Fill half a loaf pan with the stew. Top with the blended cauliflower. Drizzle with ghee or broth. Bake at 175°C (350°F) for 30 minutes.

Carrot Mousse Pudding or Cake

Ingredients:

7	large carrots, steamed until soft (5–10 minutes)
125 mL (½ cup)	butter, ghee, or coconut oil, softened
⅓ cup	honey (use progressively less as you proceed on the program)
7.5 mL (1½ tsp)	powdered ginger
¾ tsp	nutmeg
2.5 mL (½ tsp)	salt
2	large eggs, beaten

Blend all of the above until smooth and fluffy (an immersion blender will work fine). Optional: Stir 125 mL (½ cup) shredded coconut in or sprinkle it on top. As a pudding, enjoy as is. For a cake, pour into a pie plate or an 8 inch × 8 inch baking pan. Bake uncovered at 150°C (300°F) for 50–60 minutes. The result should be a moist but firm, mousse-like consistency with a slightly drier top layer. Tastiest when eaten warm.

Ghee

Put a pound of butter in a glass baking pan (a loaf pan is perfect). Heat it at 120°C (250°F) for 40–60 minutes. Three layers will form. With a shallow cooking spoon, ladle and throw out the top layer. Rinse the spoon. Ladle the middle layer (this golden liquid is the ghee) into a jar. Pour the bottom layer (white) into the garbage. Refrigerate.

More Recipes for Intro and Beyond

New to the program? Bored with your own tried and true? Whether you prefer online or hardcopy sources, there are copious options for recipes. Fans of curried, mild, sweet, light, raw, simple, or fancy will find their needs addressed. On the *Support for You* page at the GAPSguide.com website is a link to hundreds of free recipes available online, free and low-cost e-books, hardcopy books, and more. The recipes range from easy to complex, simple to layered, ingredient-abundant to ingredient-restricted (e.g., egg, dairy, or nut-free). Many are painstakingly created, tested, and posted—very often at no charge whatsoever to the reader.

To additionally ease your efforts, menu plans are also available. Some of the folks who develop recipes or menu plans can also assist with developing personalized versions for diets restricted even within the GAPS protocol.

People with limited Internet access or inclination, or those who simply prefer to work with a recipe book they can hold, might choose a hardcopy option. The only GAPS-specific hardcopy recipe book available at the time of this writing is *Internal Bliss*, available through International Nutrition (www.nutrivene.com or www.gapsdiet.com). This wonderful book was developed collaboratively by some of GAPS' tastiest bloggers, among others! Coil-bound, it presents simple, 100% GAPS-friendly instructions for preparing ingredients, as well as over 140 recipes for delicious soups, stews, main dishes, salads, appetizers, mains, breads, crackers, desserts, drinks, and (as of its most recent printing) fermentations—no adaptations required! My household has absolutely savoured the dishes found within it. Other wonderful hardcopy recipe sources which would require just a bit of attention and tweaking for GAPS (e.g., using honey in place of agave or omitting baking soda) include, but are not limited to, *The Gluten-Free Almond Flour Cookbook* by Elana Amsterdam, *The Primal Blueprint Cookbook* by Mark Sisson, and the *Grain-Free Gourmet* books by Jodi Bager and Jenny Lass. Check your local or online bookstore, or ask your local library to get them in. At any point, ask your online support group for recipe ideas and resources specific to your stage and/or individual restrictions. Finally, almost any recipe you currently have can be adapted for GAPS.

Note: When using a recipe, regardless of the source, quickly double-check each one to ensure its ingredients and preparation styles are a match for GAPS and for the stage you are on. All of us developing GAPS recipes are doing so often on the basis of conflicting or changing information. Also, it is quite easy to make an error in creating or categorizing any recipe, and even more so when working within the gentle nuances of GAPS!

In case it is a comfort to you, I will tell you that pre-GAPS, I cooked brown rice perfectly and pretty much nothing else remotely well. I'm not kidding when I tell you that just one year before the first edition of *GAPS Guide* was published, I would stand in my kitchen, burst into tears in overwhelm and stress, then walk back out, no food in hand. Learning to prepare almost 100% of our foods from scratch was a tremendous struggle for me, but I shortly got the hang of it and now whip up dishes by sense and create recipes for others! If I can, you can, too!

CHAPTER 17
MORE STORIES

Note: Because they did not yet know about it, the first two families quoted here did not implement Intro. Intro helps establish more rapid healing and allows for challenging foods to be reintegrated significantly earlier than they otherwise might.

Kevin (started modified GAPS at age 11)

"Kevin lacked oxygen at birth, so in the first year of life, I already saw that he was not developing like my other kids (he is our fifth). His motor skills lagged and he cried a lot, didn't sleep so well, etc. At two, his behaviour was just not right. He never responded right to correction, would throw things in anger or frustration, cried all the time, especially when waking up, basically never happy. He didn't walk until two and then he would fall down constantly. He also began to always be starving. When he was really hungry, his face would get distorted and frozen in a strange way. I now think he was having seizures of sorts. We did not vaccinate at all and we figured out that if we fed him lots of protein-type foods, like meats, he would relax his body and face and be able to go play for a bit until it happened all over again in a short time. I do think that because we didn't vaccinate and figured out to keep feeding him this way, we were able to "coast along" like this for years. He had learning disabilities, lacked social skills, and continued to have autistic traits like sensory issues, hiding under blankets, reacting to sounds, not liking people around, rigid in routines, and spinning and going on his head along with head banging.

"Long story shorter, we did get a diagnosis of Asperger's at one point. We took him to doc after doc, specialist after specialist to no avail. He also, strangely, was never once sick (we later learned that his immune system was not working a bit). At nine years old he got pneumonia, followed by asthma and allergies. His eating had escalated to the point of feeding him every 20–30 minutes or he would have gigantic meltdowns. We eventually could not even have people over. He was given an inhaler for the asthma and suddenly, without us making the connection, he began to not respond when called, became extremely hyperactive, and began to run away at all hours of the day and night requiring police to find him and being very dangerous (we once lost him in the middle of downtown Chicago). He would also try to jump out of moving vehicles, out of windows, and required constant restraining. The seizures got bad, he would fall down the stairs and lose consciousness several times per day. They tried psych drugs and he almost died twice from his reaction to them (I am now grateful that we couldn't go that route). We became so desperate that we brought him home from hospital and got deadbolts to keep him from running, did all our own restraining, and called alternative docs to help us.

"We began kefir and diet from nutritionist (basically a Body Ecology Diet/GAPS version), took him off inhaler. His allergies were totally out of control, he could barely open his eyes from swelling, and his chin was deformed and swollen, his belly too, his whole body. He would only eat junk food and fast foods and it was incredibly difficult to transition him to the diet. The DAN (Defeat Autism Now) protocols we followed made him worse in lots of ways because the chelation made him extremely violent, the B_{12} shots kept him awake for nights on end without any sleep, the antifungals and all those other interventions were nightmarish for him.

"Eventually, I resolved to use only foods and do this without any kind of docs. So for this past year, I researched and researched and was determined to bring him back from this state. We have done a combo of GAPS and BED very successfully along with lots of fermented foods and drinks.

"The allergies and asthma are 100% gone, the seizures we have had only one in 65 days and very mild (compared to five to ten per day). He sings every morning and has cried once in the last 2½ months (he used to cry for one to three hours at a time each day) and he can go outside again without running away. He is in martial arts, acting appropriately at church, having eye contact, no autistic traits of late and learning academics after two years of not being able to open a book. He reads before bed at an 8th grade level. It is a total absolute miracle to which I give God all the credit (there has been endless prayer at our house). I know He led us to this diet and this recovery.

"I am still fearful of regression (it's so hard to believe it's for real, you know) and I also fully realize that it will be possibly two more years before he is fully detoxed. The rashes he has had have been monumental and scary and he would have terrible seizures when the detox and die-off was going too quickly.

"I think we still have a lot to learn and a lot of work to do but there seems to be a light at the end of our tunnel. I think this is a very powerful diet and detox protocol and it really does work. I feel there is much hope and healing and we are giving our kids an opportunity at a life and future."

Two Girls (Ages 7 and 9, on GAPS for One Year)

"I have two girls, now ages seven and almost nine. Both have been dairy intolerant since weaning (thick snotty nose, sores under lip from nasal drip, and not feeling well with dairy). They could tolerate raw goat's milk, so they drank that for several years. Then they started to react to that as well, and we had to go totally dairy-free. I switched them to things made with almond milk. My younger daughter starting having a host of ills starting around when she was four: migraine-type headaches almost daily, stomachaches, unstable mood, and just feeling sick regularly. She spent way too much time on the couch, in front of the TV, because she just didn't feel well.

"Somewhere in there we put her on GF (I had gone GF for my health and found that I was very gluten intolerant). She improved greatly, but still had symptoms at times. We couldn't eat out (even GF) without her getting sick. She couldn't share snacks. I was neurotic about gluten contamination of everything. And she still wasn't really well. She also has had mild non-specific learning troubles. She was at the bottom of her class in reading. She just couldn't seem to remember the words, even from one page of the book to the next. My older daughter seemed pretty well until the summer after first grade, although in hindsight she had some symptoms before that I just didn't recognize as symptoms. By the end of the first grade summer, though, she was very ill with stomachaches daily, headaches, she was not gaining weight, and had dropped from the 85th percentile when she was two or three, to the 27th percentile. She was pale, had dark circles, was clingy, cried a lot, and was just miserable. So, we put her on GF, too. She, too, improved, but was still not really well. She, too, was near the bottom of her class in reading and cried almost nightly over math homework. Addition just seemed to escape her. We then spent months trying to eliminate this food allergen, and then that food allergen, looking for what else was making our kids not feel well. I learned to cook all kinds of different allergen-free foods, but still they were no better.

"A year ago I learned about GAPS and asked the kids if they wanted to try it. They felt miserable enough that they both said yes and we started immediately. The first several months were up and down. I'd see signs of improvement, and then something would flare and it would feel like the diet wasn't working. It was hard to judge progress because progress was so slow for us. We didn't start with Intro because no one was really promoting Intro then, so I didn't know about it. By early spring, I introduced dairy (which they hadn't had for years). My older daughter had a reaction, but my younger one didn't. A month later I tried my older daughter again, and she did fine. They both now eat lots of kefir and yogurt, both cow and goat, all raw and fermented. We have been able to add back in cheese.

"As the months have rolled by, their symptoms have faded. They have gained weight and my older daughter is now no longer bony. My younger daughter has taken off with reading, and is now solidly in the middle of the classroom pack with her reading abilities. She is a whiz in math. My older daughter, who struggled with addition, is learning multiplication and division with ease, and without any tears. Instead of watching TV because they feel ill, they ride horses, take tennis lessons, play on a soccer team, ride bikes, roller blade, etc. Our TV is almost never on anymore.

"I never got them to drink juice. I tried several times and finally gave that up. They do like freshly squeezed OJ and grapefruit juice sometimes. They drink the vegetable medley juice with meals (with mild complaints), they still take Bio-Kult, but just maintenance dose. I make them eat kraut with dinner (they hate this the most). They are still Full GAPS day in and day out, but we are venturing slowly into the world of cheating occasionally. I made a chocolate souffle for Christmas dinner which had no sugar (just honey) and was GAPS-legal except for the chocolate. They loved it and did not react.

"We started using the far infrared sauna with them a few months ago to aid detox. That has helped. Our younger daughter who was so gluten intolerant snuck a fistful of cookies once, about six months into the diet, and didn't react physically, although her reading regressed for a few weeks afterwards. This was an early sign to me that they were really healing. That sort of lapse in the past would have meant a long bout with headaches and stomachaches. I think *S. boulardii* was critical to their healing. They had a huge detox with it, and then had a huge improvement in symptoms.

"My younger daughter has been totally symptom-free for many months now. My older daughter still feels great and acts great, but wakes with the dark circles under her eyes. By mid-morning they are cleared. My older daughter complains occasionally about the diet, and pushes to have more foods added. My younger daughter never says anything about it one way or the other. It is just the way she eats; I don't think she views it as a diet. I am fearful of adding sugar or grains, so we plug along as we are. I think if they can have chocolate now and again that will buy me more time before they ask for more.

"Hope this helps. GAPS, for us at least, has not been a quick fix, and I have had periods of being discouraged and feeling like we were getting nowhere. But now that we are largely out the other side, I am so grateful to have found this diet. I feel like it has given my kids their childhoods back. For those who complain about the cooking, I can say I would rather cook than try to console my crying kid who has had a headache for days. And now my daughters help me in the kitchen. By themselves, they made Daddy and I breakfast in bed for Christmas morning, including pancakes made with almond flour."

Noah and Micah (4+ Months on GAPS)

"We have been on the diet for almost five months and are seeing huge gains. My son was diagnosed with Asperger's in May of 2008. Since then I have looked for remedies to help with hyperactivity, no focus, tantrums, anger issues, hypoglycemia, possible seizures, leg cramps, and other problems he had been having. GAPS has been a Godsend remedy for us!! It is actually working. I had to modify some things, but all and all, it's producing miracles for us!! Now we still can't have the following items: nuts, beans, any kind of fruit (throws him into hypoglycemic conditions), and also any sweet squash. Apparently, his yeast flares if he eats the squash, and he also has major problems regulating his sugar levels. I think his body has problems processing sugars, so we just avoid them and he does much better.

"I have noticed now that he is on GAPS that he isn't hungry all the time; I think this was from his body not processing his foods correctly, so his blood sugar would rise too fast and then crash. It has taken me about four years to figure this out, but I think that I have!

"Here are some of the positives: less hyperactivity, less explosive expressive language, more focus, spontaneous conversations with others, picking up on social cues better, more appropriate conversations, more empathy for others, reasoning and logic skills are improving, abstract reasoning seems to be improving, more appropriate play, more imaginative play, more engaged with his sister, less ritualistic behaviours, less echolalia and scripting, better digestion, taking naps now, better sleep at night, no more leg cramps, firm stools, and better control of his emotions…and the list could go on!!"

Your Story

As you proceed through the program, your life will become your next and all-time favourite success story! Reading and reviewing this Guide, and connecting with folks on one of the e-mail support lists, will help you navigate this path. Do not be discouraged by setbacks—they are part of the process, natural, and experienced by all of us. Your commitment to the journey will bring you rewards greater than you can even anticipate right now. It is my hope that this Guide will make the path that much easier for you than it was for those of us who did not have it. I wish you and your loved ones boundless health and happiness!

INDEX

Made in the USA
Middletown, DE
05 July 2017